AF255491

TANTRIC SEX

A BEGINNERS GUIDE WITH TANTRIC SEX POSITIONS FOR AN INCREDIBLE LIFE. EROTIC PLEASURE WITH SECRET KAMA SUTRA POSITIONS

CONTENTS

Introduction

Chapter 1:What is Tantric Sex?

Chapter 2:Description & Benefits of Tantric Sex

Chapter 3:Preparation & Teachings for Tantric Sex

Chapter 4:Tantric Sex Is Better Than the Sex You're Having

Chapter 5:Mind-Blowing Techniques of Tantric Sex

Chapter 6:Sexual Arousal and Excitement

Chapter 7:Tantric Massage, Meditation And Yoga

Chapter 8:Tantric Sex Position

Chapter 9:Tantric Erotic Massage

Chapter 10:Kama Sutra Sexual Handbook

Chapter 11:Sex In Pregnancy

Conclusion

Introduction

Imagine if you could make love with your partner for hours on end. To be intimate and connect in a way you never have before. Sex has always been a vital part of life, and it's no secret that quality sex has been linked to numerous health benefits. Lower levels of blood pressure, greater intimacy, minimized stress, happiness, and more. It is a way of reigniting the spark in the relationship.

Studies indicated that relationship happiness and well-being were attributed to not just the act of sex alone, but the affection between couples that follows after a couple has been intimate with each other, and that's just normal sex. Tantric sex? Well, that's going to revolutionize your sex life.

Before we begin exploring the emotional and cultural side of tantric sex, let's begin by first understanding the concept that tantra entails. Its practice can be traced back to ancient India, and it is a practice that many holy men and several saints used to engage in when practicing various meditational and ritualistic techniques. The term tantra is based on the metaphorical action of 'weaving' and implies the interweaving traditions and teachings as threads into a technique and or practice. While much has been written, the subject of tantra remains an elusive and mysterious thing for many who have not yet discovered its true benefits.

Tantric sex is going to challenge the beliefs you've had about sex all this time. How? Well, for one thing, the ultimate goal of tantric sex is not to achieve an orgasm. Yes, you read that right. The goal is NOT to achieve an orgasm. It teaches you to cherish your body, mind, and spirit, to treat it lovingly like the sacred vessel that it is, and to be expressive in a healthy manner. It doesn't just teach you to connect with yourself, your emotions, and your energies, but also to connect with those of your partner.

Instead, tantric sex is about transmuting your energies into higher forms. It is about the flow of your energies through your body's chakras, stimulating your sexual energy, and building on that sexual tension in your body. It takes a while, but after several weeks your body will start to experience inner peace and clarity as more of your chakras begin to open. Practitioners of tantra use it as a way of clearing the energy blocks within their bodies by fully embracing the sexual aspect of it all. The bliss that you experience during a tantric sex session helps to clear your mind. The path towards a more peaceful existence, a life where you find yourself feeling happy and fulfilled, suddenly becomes that much clearer. In short, tantric sex brings sexual freedom. It is the true meaning of what sexual freedom is all about. Orgasm may not be the ultimate goal, but don't worry because if you do it right, an orgasm is inevitable. The mind and body connection between you and your partner is going to be so powerful there's nowhere to go but towards an orgasm.

What is Tantric Sex?

Tantric sex is a type of sexual practice that stresses the spirituality of the union between a man and a woman as a sacred act. Tantric sex is about getting in touch with your sexual energy which is considered the essence of life and creation and using that energy. When you are able to tap into the energy you can have better sex and you can have sex for longer periods of time but that energy will also give you more energy in other areas of your life. It will deepen the relationship that you have with your partner because the two of you will be bonded in a spiritual and sacred way.

Tantric sex focuses on building sexual energy and then releasing it at the right time so that both of you are energized as a result. The more aware you are during sex the better the sex will be. That's why many Tantric sex rituals focus on things like touching and eye contact that are designed to make you more aware of your own energy and your partner's energy. The more deeply you can connect with your partner during Tantric sex the deeper your bond will be.

Some Tantric rituals might seem strange or awkward to you at first but once you start to practice them more you will realize that the rituals are helping you get more in touch with your own sexuality and your partner's sexuality. The rituals will help you both explore deeper and more meaningful sexual practices together which will make the relationship between you stronger.

If you have been married for a long time or if you have been with your current partner a long time and the romance has fizzled in the relationship because of kids, stress, work or other common factors exploring these Tantric sex rituals together will remind you both of why you got together in the first place. That spark between you isn't gone, it's just gotten dimmer. Tantric sex can make that spark a full burning flame of passion again.

History

Tantra the root word of tantric, means a technique to broaden consciousness. It is not a religion or philosophy. While it is based on metaphysical concepts, it is an empirical tool for those looking to create additional meaning in their lives. Furthermore, it is a technique that is based on experience, in the context of concrete life. The practice of the tantric practices is to broaden awareness in the many aspects of one's life and precisely to broaden awareness during the sexual act. In Tantra there is a joining between what often seems like opposite dimensions of pleasure and liberation. In this practice, it is the hedonistic desires that allows a person to reach a mystical experience and widen their awareness. In the Guhyasamaja Tantra it states that, "no one can achieve liberation if he engages in difficult and tormenting practices; liberation can only be achieved through the conscious fulfillment of all desires."

In addition to Tantra's creation of a bridge between sexuality and spirit, the Tantra seeks to join the concepts of both control and ecstasy. For example, in yoga the goal is to learn both self-control and discipline by removing the self through meditation. For Christians it is important to abandon oneself through self-denial and suffering, for the divine. However, in tantra both the self and the divine join each other by embracing the fulfillment of one's desires.

To briefly discuss the history of the Tantrism it is important to understand that this is a brief overview and there are many more in depth books on the history and development of the practice. Additionally, there are many books that seek to interpret Tantric texts from an ethnological, historical, cultural, religious, metaphysical and other points of view.

Around 2000 BC the Harappan populated the Hindu valley region. During this time the population, known as the Harappan society, a matriarchy, was enamored with the arts. The main concern of their society was for the well-being and each of their homes had at least one bathroom which was practically unheard of in ancient peoples of that time. The society had a major building in their capital Mohenjo-Daro. What is unique about their major building is that it was not a center of commerce or government but a swimming pool. What else is unique about this culture was that women maintained a place of honor both in their religion and secular life. She is commonly depicted with her arms open and her legs spread apart, offering herself to adoration.

It is also worth noting the use of the Harappan, to lay a large bed in the main room of the houses. It was the bed of the landlady, and there – in the main room, in the living room – the act of love was celebrated.

In this society religion was a daily practice. It was not just a system of dogmatic doctrine but an experience where the divine was personal to the practitioner. For the Harrapan religion was closely connected with the body, pleasure, and sexuality. This is in contrast to more patriarchal societies where the divine was far away from the practitioners. For patriarchal religious communities there became a need to bridge the space between man and their god or gods which required the use of rituals and holy people. When their society eventually transitioned to becoming more male centered the religious beliefs undertook a change.

For those that practice Tantra they know that there is a wide range of female representation. This is in contrast to the Christian centered culture where being female is broken and a woman is both clean and chaste or a dirty whore. However, in Tantrism female representations can both sexual and spiritual, ecstatic and intelligent, fierce and peaceful. They can be spiritual without denying who they are as women.

Tantrism enjoyed a great increase in followers in the period between 10th and 12th centuries AD. However, it was later suppressed with the introduction of Islam to the region. During this time there were secret schools of Tantrism that survived in places like Bengal and Assam where they had good relationships with China. Part of this was because of the beliefs on sexuality that Taoists had. In contrast, in places like Tibet where they were sheltered from the influence of other societies Tantrism flourished and married with the ideas espoused in Buddhism and Bon. Bon is an ancient shamanic religion.

The Spread of Tantrism

In 8th century AD, the Guru Padmasambhava, a famous Indian tantric, traveled to Tibet. In the 11th century, Tibetan translator Marpa traveled to India to study Tantra da Naropa, a disciple of Tilopa. When Marpa returned to Tibet he translated and taught the Tantric principles to his famous disciple Milarepa. From this period began the widespread dissemination of Tantra in Tibet. It is because of Milarepa that in women are revered and considered wise after to males.

Over time there began a distancing of the sexual practices of Tantrism to a different form. This form of less sexually charged Tantrism is called Red Tantra or Tantra of the Left Hand. It is about studying the union of men and women on the level of their energy. There is also a more metaphysical concept of Tantrism that is called White Tantra or Tantra of the Right Hand.

These newer forms of Tantra lend to the Buddhist mantra that is loosely translated as "the jewel in the lot." For them the jewel is the male organ and the lot is the lotus flower or the female sexual organ. They can come together in both the physical and mystical sense.

After this followed a series of years of decline for Tantra in India. However, it was with the start of the sexual revolution of the 1970s and the women's liberation movement that there was a rediscovery of the Tantric arts. It was during this time that many of the Tibetan llamas and Hindu yogis opened their teachings to Westerners. Two of the many yogis and llamas charged with the spread of White Tantra to the west are Llama Yesce and Yogi Bhajan who gave Westerners more up-to-date and understandable texts. Teaching these old techniques to a new audience did not happen easily. One of the major problems was translating the texts and reading the instructions without breaking up the energy. However, after much efforts were made these problems much easier to deal with. However, there were things like sayings in the text that were left up for interpretation. Another barrier to its adoption in the west were the learning of the many different poses that could be used in the practice of Tantra.

However, with the increase of sexuality in both men and women and the liberation of women from the traditional female roles sex has become more enjoyable for the masses and has allowed many to understand the Tantric arts. However, it is important to understand that the adoption of Tantra has had nothing to do with this liberation and more to do with the enjoyment and pleasure of sex seen in many today. People in today's culture now see sex as an obligation and it must always be good sex. However, Tantra reminds us that it is not the same as Tantric sex. Tantric sex seeks to find ecstasy and liberation in the sexual act and not as the end means of all sexual contact.

The purpose of Tantric sex is not to find enjoyment in the sex act in and of itself but to find a spiritual experience in the joining of the male and female.

For those in Western society the use of Tantra is two-fold. It is used to first, draw a spiritual map that connects us with the larger dimensions of the self in a very practical and experiential sense; and second to create a culture of love. In the West's culture of love the traditions are scarce and experiences have to be made up by the practitioner themselves. However, there are some cultural events like red-light districts in European areas and gentlemen's or strip clubs that are part of the culture of eroticism. However, for these red-light districts and strip clubs the feeling generated is mostly depressing and not seen as a highlight to the sexual experience.

In the West, there tends to be an overload of sexual messages of every kind both images and words. However, while it seems that everything is permissible it has not yet extended to the real-life bedrooms of the men and women that are living in the society. All of the sexual needs and energy, in the West, is reserved for the fantasy realm and not real life. This is in contrast to those practitioners of the tantric arts who create concrete situations with a high erotic charge. These practitioners are doing so based on the belief that this is a spiritual ritual that happens to involve sex. The sex is part of the spiritual experience and is not reserved solely for the mind and a hidden drawer of the room.

In tantra the sexual ritual is called pancha-makara. Also known as the five "M"s. The five Mems are madya or drink wine, mamsa or eat meat, matsya eat fish, mudra or eat an aphrodisiac cereal, and maithuna or join sexually. However, in vegetarian societies these "M"s were modified to be considerate of the values espoused in that society. However, these other five M rituals do not seem to have the same value in a culture where meat, fish, and wine are available at the push of an app or in any corner store or supermarket at a moment's notice. However, the idea is clearly to enjoy life and the sustenance that surrounds it including the sexual act which is just as important for Tantric followers as eating or drinking. It is important to remember that at the time of the Tantra's original writing those things, meat, fish, wine, and even sex were not easily taken for granted and were seen in a scarcity and something to savor and enjoy as part of the enjoyment of a life.

It is with this that many of the Tantric schools have started to re-emphasize the importance of the other four "M"s not just the one that involves sex. They have done this because of the age of indulgence that we live in to help people become more serene and pleased in what they may see as the doldrums of food and beverage in a society over flowing with sustenance. They have developed many of the rituals to be more sustainable by modern practitioners in a more modern world. They want the practitioners to understand that Tantra is not a hedonistic orgy of food, wine and sex but a ritual that uses sex and food as a way to reach deep into the heart and find a spirituality in it.

Origins

Now, that you know the basic etymology of 'Tantra' let us dive right in and get more information as to the origins and the history of this rather misunderstood and misinterpreted system of thought. Tantra can be believed to be the weaving of the 'sutras' of Siva and that of Shakti to achieve the divine and transcend beyond human senses. There were multiple oral traditions that were imbibed into the Tantra of weaving together of Siva and Shakti. These traditions were most likely derived from Dravidian matriarchal societies that honored and respected the female aspect of life. In these traditions, women were very powerful influencers and great teachers too.

There were highly powerful and meaningful rituals to mark transition points. These rituals were all centered upon nature and were very important connecting lines to nature. Most importantly, these female-oriented traditions rarely separated these rituals from routine life. They did not have priestly class or any kind of monastic order which controlled the other parts of the society or tradition.

These teachings or the Tantra thoughts found a lot of popularity among the burgeoning middle class in India, which was becoming wealthier and more powerful than before the time we are talking about (around the 6th century). This emerging middle class was more or less unaffected by the caste-consciousness of the Vedic nature and also by the monastic male-dominated Buddhist philosophy of the times.

Additionally, these shamanic-like traditions taught that enlightenment was possible right here, right now. These traditions were practical and easy to follow unlike the scholarly and monastic teachings of the conventional religions in force at that time. These traditions were very immediate and very vibrant too.

The immediacy of the outcomes was very attractive as people did not have the compulsion to wait for reincarnations and rebirths for salvation. Divinity was not described in any abstract and distant form consisting of a collection of confusing deities. On the other hand, divinity was explained as something that is all-pervasive and that which each of us is a part of. In fact, divinity is not something that we are a part of, but it was the whole of the Universe.

Nothingness, as described in Buddhism, this was not an easy concept to understand for the average person. The concept of nothingness was changed into a form that was easier to interpret and comprehend; that nothingness became an all-pervading, omnipresent, and universal consciousness.

The physical world which was considered a deception to the traditional view became an illusion in this middle-class accepted new tradition. Everything and everyone in this universe became a differently projected part of the universal consciousness. As we get better at understanding, the awareness of the non-duality concept, we slowly began to understand the illusionary aspect of what our five senses project to us until finally, we can now visualize and accept the entire Universe including us, the world around us, and the Divine, as one and the same.

All these teachings together were referred to as Tantra and continued through the entire Classical Era, which lasted for about 400-500 years. Multiple individual and independent teachers created many lineages that had among them a few diversities but mostly commonalities.

Kashmir Shaivism was one such lineage created and remained highly prevalent for a few centuries. However, the Tantra lineage highly influenced both the then prevalent Hinduism and Buddhism. The Hinduism as we know it today is particularly influenced by the Tantra tradition. Buddhism created an entirely new sub-sect called Vajrayana Buddhism that still survives in the Himalayas even today.

Description & Benefits of Tantric Sex

Tantra, translated from Sanskrit to mean "tools for expansion", is essentially a set of practices and instructions designed to connect us with our inner energy and emotions, thereby allowing us to become more aware of the energy around us. Tantra encourages us to explore sexual energy to meet these ends.

Tantra is actually a system to help you achieve a higher plane of consciousness, referred to as Samadhi. The use of sex is only an instrument to achieve this Samadhi state. The actual act of sex is designed to take you beyond carnal pleasures that are limited to human senses. While the pleasure aspect of sex is also heightened through the use of tantric practices, these practices are also helpful in improving your physical and spiritual health.

There are usually two paths of Tantric practices that are used; the left-hand path and the right-hand path. For the average person, the left-hand path is considered most appropriate as it helps in achieving tantric enlightenment without sacrificing sexual pleasure. The right-hand path is more for the highly advanced practitioner and may not suit the needs of the average beginner. The processes in the right-hand path focus on intense meditative and symbolic techniques connected to sexual energy but without participating in the actual sexual act itself. Both these paths are 'correct' and it is not possible to say which is better than the other.

Tantra principles are based on a presumption that sexual energy comes from the base chakras including:

- Muladhara chakra

- Svadhisthana chakra

- Manipura chakra

All the above chakras are located either at the navel level or below it. This sexual energy originating from the base chakras can be moved up to the upper chakras which are:

- Anahata or the heart chakra

- Visuddha or the throat chakra

- Anja or the third eye chakra

- Sahasrara or the crown chakra

The deliberate movement of the sexual energy from the base chakras to the upper chakras through tantric practices and rituals is designed to enhance both sexual and spiritual experience for the practitioners. The benefits include more fulfilling and more sustaining outcomes of both the sexual and spiritual experiences than before.

The tantric practices not only gives enhanced and the ultimate sexual pleasure that all of us strive to achieve but also benefits our physical and spiritual growth. The tantric practices, if done correctly and as per set norms, will help in producing sensations of bliss through love and sexual union from the human perspective and also from the perspective of joining the male and female energies through the act.

In the commonly practiced sexual encounters, most of the participants voice a sense of dissatisfaction and incompletion from the act in addition to feeling exhausted after reaching sexual peaks. This rather debilitating feeling of exhaustion is not just temporary but can easily spill over into other aspects of your emotional and physical life leaving you tired and fatigued more often than you'd like.

The loss of life energy or prana is bound to lead to health imbalances that can ultimately lead you to not enjoy the act at all. Using a few asanas, yoga postures, and some techniques from the teachings of Tantra, it is possible for a couple to preserve sexual energy and direct it upwards making sure every cell in the body is awakened through these practices.

For example, there is a technique referred to as transfiguration in tantra in which a couple sit in front of each other (fully clothed) without any physical contact and gaze into each other's eyes. It is important not to reduce this technique to a mere staring exercise. This tantric exercise requires you to be with your partner in a very intimate and profound way. By following this practice diligently, you will notice that there will come a time when both of you can see a personality beyond the eyes.

Each of you will see a certain beauty in the other that is impossible to ignore, reject or hate. Finding this almost pure enigma in each other will create a kind of love in the relationship that will go beyond human expectations and requirements from the each other allowing for free love to flow between the partners resulting in a deeper and more connected relationship.

The benefits to practicing Tantra can be phenomenal. Some men are able to reach unlimited multiple orgasms in one encounter, as opposed to single ejaculations that signal the end of an interaction. In fact, ejaculation as an end goal of sex can possibly become obsolete because so much pleasure is experienced during the act of making love in and of itself. In this way, sex can last for several hours and the heightened emotional, physical and spiritual connection between lovers is amplified.

However, the goal of Tantric sex is not necessarily to achieve orgasm, but rather to enrich the entire sexual encounter by allowing us to experience more variety and depth in our sexuality.

Frequently, Western approaches to improving our sex lives encourage us to evaluate and alter external components of ourselves and our lives. For example, we are constantly told through advertisements (frequently through sexual imagery) that we will be happier and more attractive, and, therefore, will have more fulfilling lives if we would just lose weight, gain muscle, drive a nicer car or buy a better perfume or cologne. Tantric sex, in contrast, ignores all of those external, materialistic characteristics and encourages us to become better lovers and better partners, thus achieving more fulfilling sexual experiences through reciprocity of intention and desire to please.

Some have reported being able to come to orgasm by simply looking at and thinking about the object of their affection -- touching is optional. Still others have become so skilled in the art of Tantra that they have led completely fulfilled sex lives going months at a time without ejaculating, even while having sex every single day!

The more a person -- be they male or female -- engages in sex but refrains from ejaculating, the more energy they retain as opposed to experiencing the loss of energy that regularly occurs (especially for men) when ejaculate is released. After Tantric sex, people report experiencing more energy and vitality and couples describe overall increased satisfaction with the duration, intensity and quality of their sex lives.

Physical Benefits

Here are some of the physical benefits reported by practitioners of Tantra-based techniques driven by increased and seamless energy flow through the bloodstream into every nook and corner of the body:

- Improved toning of muscles
- Rejuvenated and revitalized skin texture leading to improved complexion
- Reduced movement of the spinal cord and slow back pain
- Reduction in fat deposits
- Release of toxins from the body
- Maintenance of youthful energy and looks along with improved physical vitality
- Reduction in wrinkles
- Firmer breasts
- Toning of muscles in the hip and the abdomen resulting in a flatter tummy and improved gait quality
- Calf muscles were highly regenerated

- A sustained sense of joy and happiness
- Reduction in menstrual secretions along with reduced premenstrual symptoms

Men practitioners also reported increased benefits from the preservation and redirection of sexual energy resulting in a healthier body and improved creative energy flow throughout the system. Tantra practices encourage the consumption of a low-protein macrobiotic diet that has a balanced amount of yin and yang to match the feminine and masculine balance resulting from following tantric practices.

Women practitioners are highly benefited as well as Tantra practices help in building and improving overall general health by channelizing the preserved energy right through the body. Tantra techniques help to calm the body and mind while improving energy levels. Practicing tantra techniques is a way for people to retreat themselves from this mad, hectic world and re-energize their body and mind. Especially, through the regular practice of Tantra yoga asanas which call for steady and slow movements of the body moving from one asana to another seamlessly. The conscious breathing done during this time is always a method to calm down your mind.

More Benefits of Tantric Sex

Tantric sex will help in bringing two people closer together and help in their spiritual, emotional and mental union.

Individual Growth

Tantric sex helps in increasing the intimacy quotient in a relationship. It also helps in the growth of individuals as well. A person would be able to grow mentally, physically, as well as spiritually. Tantric sex helps in awakening Kundalini in women, and this allows for her feminine nature to shine through. She will start to glow and have a more positive outlook and attitude towards life. The male energy, Shiva helps a man to harness all his masculine energy through peace and inner strength.

Exploring the Limits

Quickies and self-pleasuring techniques are becoming quite common these days, and people are more often than not missing out on the benefits that meaningful and loving sex can provide. This hinders an individual from exploring their sexual limits. Tantric sex can help turn this around. Tantric sex would help an individual in understanding their true sexuality and their sexual limits. When a couple engages in Tantric sex, they form a deep and meaningful bond that allows each partner to experience sexual bliss. Tantric sex can be thought of like a team effort where each partner helps the other reach and reel in great physical, emotional and sexual pleasure that can be experienced by both.

Heightened Orgasms

The orgasms achieved through Tantric sex are more powerful than the ordinary ones. The various tantric sex positions mentioned in this book will help you in achieving earth-shattering orgasms. The positions are designed such that they hit all the sweet spots and make your body sing. It is a general notion that women can have a higher level of orgasm when compared to men, but with Tantric sex, both men and women can achieve a higher state of orgasm.

Knowing What Works

Once you have managed to get the hang of it, Tantric sex can be enjoyable and exciting. With each successive session, you will get a better understanding of your sexuality, your triggers and also those of your partner. You will be able to understand what you and your partner enjoy. Once you have managed to identify these pleasure points, you can start stimulating them for achieving pure sexual bliss. The physical and mental bond that you would have established with your partner would simply depend on him and strengthen over a period and you will reach a stage where you, as a couple, become dependent on each other's sexual energy for their pleasure.

Timed Bliss

You can time your orgasms with Tantric sex. Once an individual has managed to gain control over their mind as well as body, they can automatically fall into a synchronized pattern for attaining a mutual orgasm. A new form of energy is generated, and it flows through each of them when they have timed orgasms. This does amplify the bond between couples. Teachings of Tantric sex suggest that staying connected after a sexual act will help in strengthening the bond that's formed.

Monogamy

It is a popular belief that Tantric sex can help a couple in staying together for the rest of their lifespan. When two individuals have managed to forge a bond that helps them to connect on a deeper plane, they become dependent. This dependency cannot be mimicked or replicated with anyone else. When the frequency of the session starts to increase, then the bond between the individuals also starts to deepen and strengthen.

Health benefits

Tantric sex does help in promoting good health. Women will benefit from this because it will help in making their menstrual cycle more regular and this, in turn, helps them in keeping their bodies in good shape. Tantric sex helps in producing certain male hormones that produce healthier and stronger sperms, thereby increasing the couple's fertility. A full body orgasm helps in fueling the body cells and also helps in increasing their strength to combat disease, thereby increasing the immunity. Women and men who have Tantric sex tend to look younger because this is a great stress buster. It also adds a new glow to the face. Apart from all the various benefits that it has to offer everyone, Tantric sex can also help in producing serotonin that assists in keeping depression at bay. An orgasm helps in releasing serotonin that helps in keeping cortisol at bay and improves an individual's mood.

Inhibitions

It also helps in making a person get accustomed to their body and be more comfortable with their body and that of their partner. Most people in this day and age tend to get extremely conscious about their bodies and these fears that they harbor stop them from thoroughly enjoying sex and they end up having mediocre sex. Once you let go of the fear of being judged and have accepted your body for the way it is, then you will be able to truly let go and savor the moment, as it was meant to be enjoyed. If you let go of all these fears, you can enjoy physical pleasure. Letting go of your inhibitions will make sex more enjoyable. Tantric sex encourages this abandonment.

Power struggle

If you follow the popular television series "The Game of Thrones," then you will remember the episode where Daenerys Targaryen breaks all the norms and decides to take charge of pleasuring her alpha-male husband, Khal Drogo. Drogo objects at first, but then he gives in once he realizes how pleasurable it really is. When it comes to sex, more often than not, people tend to face an inner power struggle. Men and women both tend to like the feeling of being in control, through showing that they are in control can do serious damage to a relationship. There is a difference between being in control and enjoying mutual Tantric sex. Tantric sex will help in eliminating this problem altogether. Tantric sex gives equal power to both the partners and the different positions will help in allowing both the parties to be in charge and they can give each pleasure the other person without any restrictions.

Happiness

Tantric sex helps in channeling all the positive forms of energy and this will help in making the individual extremely happy. Since it is spiritually, emotionally and physically satisfying, an individual would be happy in all these aspects. The spiritual connection that it lets you form with divinity helps.

Increased love

There are thousands of thoughts that go through your mind at any given point of time. We tend to think about different people, not necessarily our partners. It's quite common these days for couples to break off their relationships on the pretext that they aren't feeling "the love" anymore. Tantric sex will not only help you in loving yourself, but it will also help you in loving your partner. It helps in developing a nurturing relationship that helps in mutual growth. This kind of strength of feeling makes the relationship more solid.

Empowers both Men and Women

Most women tend to suffer from low self-esteem. They have become plagued with thoughts and feelings that their bodies are imperfect. They may not have the power to say no to their partner while engaged in a sexual act. They may not be truly willing to have sex but are forced into it because of their inability to say no. They might not express their true feelings and desires freely, and this reduces the pleasure that they experience. According to the teachings of Tantric sex, women are treated like goddesses, and they are showered with the attention and the respect that they deserve. Likewise, even men are plagued with different issues regarding the way they perceive themselves. Most men worry about the way they are performing, whether or not they can satisfy their partner if their stamina is good enough and so on and so forth. Instead of enjoying the act, they are often worried about how long they can last. When they follow the teachings of Tantric sex, they will feel empowered since their bodies are honored as the vessels of God. This will make them more confident and open to new experiences without having to live with those fears and inhibitions.

Immense Satisfaction

There are times when you might have had sex and felt that something was missing in it. You might feel that there's no excitement or romance. This tends to happen since sex doesn't go beyond intercourse. It stops at the physical act. Sex alone does not do anything for a relationship. Tantric sex is more pleasurable since it helps in forming an emotional bond between partners instead of a simple physical bond. When a person is emotionally invested in an act, it becomes more pleasurable and enjoyable. When both are, it becomes magical.

Alleviates Depression

Think of Tantric sex as your counselor. It will help you in overcoming depression and even anxiety. People are usually too tired to eat or sleep these days. This wreaks havoc on their daily schedule. Tantric sex will help you in tackling the problems mentioned above. After a session of Tantric sex, you will feel revitalized and reenergized, and this newfound peace and energy will relax your body and calm your mind, thereby getting rid of all the unnecessary tensions that keep stressing you.

Preparation & Teachings for Tantric Sex

Prepare Your Body

The teachings of Tantric sex believe that your body is a temple of love and that it is really important that you keep in healthy. If you want to achieve higher levels of ecstasy, then you will need to keep fit. This time, you will learn about the different tips that you can make use of for keeping your body fit and healthy. There are specific yoga positions that you can make use of if you want to facilitate the movement of energy in your body. More often than not, we tend to take our bodies for granted. We don't worry about it, and we don't realize that the body is the bridge that will help you in attaining bliss. You will need to worship your body and treat it with the care and love it deserves if you want to attain a higher level of bliss.

Building love for your body through the looking glass

One of the most important things that you will need to do while you are preparing your body for Tantric sex is to let go of all the different negative thoughts that you might harbor about your body. You will have to view every part of your body, including your genitals and see whether or not they are healthy. If you feel that you are fat, simply tell yourself that you are curvy. You must do this regularly to make sure that you let go of any negative feelings that you might have towards your body and instead enjoy yourself and have fun while having sex.

When was the last time you have seen yourself naked? Try standing naked in front of a full-length mirror. You can do this after taking a shower if you prefer to do this. Take a close look at every inch of your body. Start from your feet right up to the top of your head. If you notice that you are criticizing yourself, then stop then and there and instead give yourself a compliment. Replace every negative thought with a positive one. If you feel that your ass is fat or that your thighs are thick, simply think that you have a luscious body! You needn't worry about what you look like. Change every negative feeling into a positive one. Then observe your genitals. You should focus on every little aspect of your genitals, the colors, shape and also the moistness in particular areas. It is really important that you do this to be confident about your body.

Teachings of Tantric Sex

Let us take a closer look at the teachings of Tantric sex that will help in not only improving the level of intimacy but also the sexual pleasure that you and your partner experience. This will have a positive effect on your relationship. When these teachings are made use of in the proper manner, then it will put you a step closer to achieving enlightenment. Each one of these teachings can be made use of in a sexual and a non-sexual way.

Breathe

Remember to keep breathing. You probably would have understood by now the importance of breathing when it comes to Tantric sex. It is not just about tantric sex; any of the teachings that have originated in the East, regarding the attainment of enlightenment, tend to place a great deal of importance on breathing. It is crucial that you understand the reason why this is done and the manner in which it is related to Tantra as well as the spiritual development of an individual.

The answer to this is quite simple, every living thing breathes. We breathe all the time, and if we do stop breathing for prolonged periods of time, it will ultimately result in death or even unconsciousness. In this manner, it could be simply understood that breathing can be related to our state of consciousness. Think of breath as energy. Every breath that we take fills our body with oxygen and takes away carbon dioxide in this process. This oxygen that we inhale is then supplied to different cells in the body. Oxygen and breathing are fundamental for the functioning of our bodies. Breathing isn't a voluntary or conscious function. It is something that our body has been designed to do. You might never pay any attention to the way you are breathing, but you never really stop breathing when you are alive. Isn't it intimidating how our life depends on a function that we don't even do voluntarily?

It is quite interesting to note the benefits of conscious and regulated breathing can have on different aspects of your life, including your sex life. It is common that while people are engaged in any sexual activity, they tend to hold their breath, this isn't a known function. Every time you get excited, you might notice that you tend to hold your breath. You probably hold onto your breath without even realizing that you are doing so. When you stop breathing, this will disrupt the flow of energy in your body as well. Making breathing a conscious act while engaged in sex will help you in learning to control your energy and the movement of energy in your body. This teaching of Tantra is all about taking breaths in a relaxed and calm manner. Let your breath flow slowly through your body. If you want to achieve a full body orgasm, then you will have to make sure that your breathing is deep and even. When you start focusing on this, you will realize that you can climax more easily.

Relax

The tension in your muscles and body will act as an obstruction in a manner that is similar to shallow breathing. The muscular tension that you tend to experience when you are engaged in any sexual activity is not a conscious one. One of the principles of Tantric sex is that you will need to be aware of this muscular tension that exists in your body and so that you are aware of all the different muscles that are being held up due to tension. You do require a little bit of tension for facilitating movement in the body and also for holding up the body, but that's it. Muscular tension isn't required in every part of the body.

If you start making the decision of tensing up your muscles a conscious one, then you will notice that you are probably tensing up a few muscles in your body unnecessarily while having sex. For instance, a man might end up tensing all his muscles while receiving oral sex. Whereas he's simply supposed to let go and enjoy the attention being showered by his partner, instead he is tensing up the muscles in his torso and legs. In such a case, all the extra tension is unnecessary, and this simply obstructs the free flow of energy in the body. Focus your attention on relaxing all these tensed muscles. Focus on your breathing and enjoy the sexual warmth that is flowing through your body.

Sounds that can help

Sounds are crucial when it comes to the movement of energy in the body. Some people may not be comfortable, or they might even be conscious about the sounds that they make when aroused. These considerations shouldn't be taken seriously while engaging in Tantric sex. Let go of all the inhibitions that are holding you back. Express yourself as freely as you want to. There is no restriction apart from the ones that you have imposed on yourself. Make all the sounds that you feel like making. These sounds are involuntary reactions to the pleasure that you are experiencing, and they are connected with the emotions and sensations that you are experiencing. If you are silent or quiet, then the movement of sexual energy in your body gets slow. When you are vocal in expressing what you are feeling, the energy starts to move in the body. Tantric sex is all about awakening the dormant sexual energy that is present within the body and then making use of it for achieving enlightenment. Well, how will the energy move when you are anxious about something as trivial as the way you sound?

Eye contact is essential

This might sound like an obvious thing. Well, it does enhance the overall sexual experience. Looking at your partner while engaged in any sexual act will make the experience more intense eye contact doesn't mean that you stare wistfully into your partner's eyes. Move over to the longing look a love struck puppy has in its eyes. We are talking about some serious X-rated gazing, so get ready for it. This will help you attain some extra intimacy. For getting started, you and your partner can find a comfortable spot to sit so that you both will be able to look into each other's eyes. Take a moment to gather your thoughts; usually, a deep breath will do the trick for you. Once you feel that you are ready, you can open your eyes and gaze into your partner's eyes. Allow your partner the access to see you, your true self, sans any pretenses and in a similar manner, you can gaze at them. This might feel a little stupid initially, but it will prove to be quite effective.

Allow yourself to communicate through your eyes and not just your genitals. You can let your eyes wander over each other's body. Let your partner see the lust in your eyes and the wanton abandonment. Nothing would be a better turn on than knowing that your partner desires you and needs you. In the manner, that sounds and touch can communicate, in the same way, you can communicate a lot more by making use of just your eyes alone. This will help you both communicate with each other in an earnest manner.

Pay attention

Energy flows in the body according to your attention. You will need to concentrate on this flow of energy in your body. If you want to experience a full body orgasm, then the energy in your body should spread to every single cell. You will have to start paying some extra attention to the highly sexualized feelings that you want to experience throughout your body. If a woman wants to enjoy a vaginal orgasm, then she will need to focus on prying out the dormant sexual energy that is present within her and coax it to move freely in her body. You can make use of the other principles of Tantra for focusing your attention. For drawing out the energy and directing it towards the spot that you want it to go to, then you will need to visualize the same. Picture this energy moving from its resting place to the place where you want to experience pleasure. The principles of Tantra suggest that energy needn't be confined to only one part of the body and that it, in fact, should be moving throughout the body.

Always be present

The basic principle of all teachings is the need to be present in the moment. Present doesn't imply being present physically. It means being present mentally as well. You will have to be present in the moment. Don't let your mind or thoughts wander anywhere and don't fantasize about anything else apart from the activity that you are involved in at the moment. Be present in the moment with your partner, and be aware of what is happening.

Exploration of your senses

Tantra is an ancient art, and it's been around for centuries. It is crucial to take note of the fact that Tantra isn't just about improving the physical quality of having intercourse, but it is also about enhancing the emotional experience. All your sensory organs tend to take part in your sexual experience. Sex isn't an isolated process. Therefore, Tantra is all about improving your sensory experience as well. If one of your senses has been compromised then, the other senses tend to become sensitive.

Aim for a full body orgasm

Who wouldn't want to have an orgasm? A full body orgasm does sound tempting, doesn't it? So, without wasting any time, let us get started with this fascinating concept. One manner in which you can condition your body to have a full body orgasm is by practicing the build up to an impending orgasm and then letting it subside without giving in to the pleasure. You will have to drive your partner to the brink of an orgasm and then let it fade away, without letting them climax. Once you let it subside, you will have to start building it up again and let it fade away again. Use all your willpower and keep playing at it for as long as you possibly can.

The journey counts

Orgasms are wonderful, but Tantric sex isn't about simply achieving an orgasm. It is about delaying your orgasm for a while longer to receive better results. An orgasm can be thought of as a wonderful by-product of engaging in Tantric sex. Tantric sex is more spiritual and sacred than regular sex. It is the union of the opposing sexual energies present in the partners. The pressure of having to achieve an orgasm tends to take away the pleasure of participating in a sexual act. This stress is quite harmful, and it has a negative impact on the person's performance. The journey in Tantric sex is almost as important as a result. Orgasm isn't the main aim. It is about enjoying your body and your partner as well. It is about worshiping each other's bodies and cherishing your time together. Sex means so much more than a mere physical act that a couple would engage in. Try shifting your focus to different things that you enjoy and also the things that your partner finds pleasurable. There will certainly be certain things that you both seem to enjoy. Find those common things. It may be kissing, foreplay, holding each other or any oral activity and incorporate these into your lovemaking process.

Tricks of Pleasure

When the emotional component is very high, any touch, kissing, licking or biting of any part of the body can result in a powerful sexual stimulation. This is because the entire body can be an erotic zone if you receive contact from someone who is sexually attractive and desirable. However, the truth is that certain parts of your body are particularly sexually sensitive. These areas are often called erogenous zones, and their sensitivity is due to the rich network of nerve terminations. In a sexual circumstance, tactile or buccal stimulation in these areas become the first step to stimulate the whole body.

The Thigh High

Select your favorite essential oil and pour a few drops of this scented oil onto your hands. Make sure that your plasma are well oiled and then place these on your partner's thighs, a little above their knee. Start by gently kneading and move upwards. Take your time and let the anticipation build. This buildup of sexual tension will just add to the experience and make it more pleasurable. Don't touch your partner's genitals; instead, focus on the areas around the genitals.

Take the Nail Road

Make use of your nails and gently trace patterns of looks eight on your lover's thigh or run your nails lightly along the length of their back or their calf. Tease all those areas that are sensitive to touch and vary the pressure to elicit different reactions from your partner.

Try the Aural Sex Rub

Take some time and try and massage your partner's ear. Make sure that you are being gentle and make use of light touches. Use your fingers and start working from the outer fold of the ear towards the inner ear. Run your little finger along the outer edge of the finger. You can whisper sweet nothings and endearments into your partner's ear while doing this. You can gently lick and poke around with your tongue if you are feeling slightly adventurous.

Now, Turn Up the Heat

After all the teasing and the tantalizing foreplay, it is time to turn up the heat. You and your partner can indulge in some oral sex or explore one of the many tantric sex. It is up to you, the manner in which you want to turn up the heat in the bedroom. Take your time as you did with all the foreplay. It isn't a quickie; it is about savoring the moment and honoring each other's bodies.

Tantric Sex Is Better Than the Sex You're Having

Reasons Why Tantric Sex is the Better Sex

There is more to tantra than meets the eye. Tantric sex is just but a single aspect of tantra, and if you're wondering why you should begin adopting this approach to sex, you'll be pleased to discover there are many reasons why. Whether you're looking to make a better connection, improve your sex life or just trying to shake up your relationship, once you set foot down this powerful sacred sexual pathway, you won't want to go back to the way it used to be.

Once you've decided to embrace tantric sex in your life, the old routines and habits need to be tossed out the window. You're beginning anew with a fresh mindset, with a focus on not just enjoying sex, but also enjoying the freedom of being able to express your pleasure. Powerful orgasms (although that isn't the main goal, mind you), orgasms that last longer, multiple orgasms, enhanced intimacy levels, and better sex life overall are some of the many wonderful benefits that await you.

- It Makes You Feel More Spiritual - Spirituality is not about being religious; it is about getting in touch with your soul and what truly matters in your life. Tantra opens you to a higher connection between you and your spiritual side. Being spiritual shifts your perspective to focus on the things that should matter most to you, leads you away from being too focused or consumed about the materialistic aspects of this world we are so often caught up with.

- It gets rid of the Pressure to "Perform" - Porn has led to a lot of misconceptions about what sex should be. Porn is not bad per se, but it can make you feel pressured to live up to those unrealistic expectations that you see on screen. We fail to remember that at the end of the day, what you see on screen is nothing more than performance. Purely for entertainment purposes. Tantra helps you eliminate some of that pressure by acting as the "anti-porn." Instead of focusing on living up to expectations, tantra slows things down with movements that teach you to appreciate being in the moment with your partner. This is someone you love, and you should take the time to show them that love. Think about this moment when it is just the two of you and no one else. Gaze lovingly into their eyes and think about all the reasons why you love them for who they are.

- It Teaches You to Accept Yourself for Who You Are - The person you are right at this moment is the person you are bringing to the tantric experience you have with your partner. Embracing yourself for you who see yourself for who you are. We may not admit it out loud; many of us are afraid of letting someone else see our true selves in case they don't like what they see. Tantra teaches you to look deep into your soul and into your heart, and because tantra is about focusing on your energy, it makes it impossible for you to hide from the truth any longer.

- It Encourages Communication - Do you listen to your partner during sex? Do they listen to you? You both will once you begin the art of tantric sex since mindfulness is a big part of making this work. It encourages you to communicate when you slow it down and talk to each other and focus on what feels good as you touch each other. Couples are encouraged to be honest and as specific as possible. As your partner touches you, think about what that sensation feels like. Does it feel good? Let them know. Would you prefer something else? Let them know. Tantric sex is about getting out of your own head and turning your attention towards your body instead.

- It Teaches You to Explore Your Limits - Self-pleasuring techniques and quickies have taken away the meaning of what a sexual experience filled with love can do for you. When you miss out on that, it hinders you from exploring your sexual limits. Tantric sex, of course, aims to turn that around by helping you understand your true sexuality. Couples who engage in tantric sex form a deep, meaningful bond, and it is this bond that allows both parties to experience sexual bliss. You work together as a team to see how far you can push your limits, how much more pleasure you can attain, and earth-shattering orgasms that follow will make your body sing like never before.

It Promotes Monogamy - A deep bond that is formed with another is a bond that is not severed quite so easily. The kind of bond that you form with your partner during tantric sex is going to transcend the connection you had previously before you began this journey. The closer you grow, the deeper your feelings become, and when you feel such love and affection for another, the desire to look elsewhere for pleasure gradually fades away.

Tantric sex is something that both men and women can benefit from. The rejuvenating effects that it has claims to bring with it several health benefits because of the way that it changes the body's chemistry. Aside from the benefits that were talked about above, tantric sex is even better than the sex you're having right now because of the individual benefits it has for men and women. There are unique ways in which men and women benefit from the art of tantric sex.

For women, tantric sex is going to nourish the body, infuse the woman with energy and touch her heart and soul completely. For women, these are the reasons why tantric sex is better sex:

- *The Health Benefits* - It empowers a woman's endocrine glands, stimulating it to produce more of the HGH hormone, more serotonin, testosterone, and even the DHEA hormone. The energy that flows throughout the woman's body during sex can help to detoxify her through each breath that she takes, even improving her cardiovascular and immune system. Breathing techniques and learning how to regulate breath alone, for example, is a way of improving your health by allowing more air into the body, which then helps to nourish all the muscles and tissue within the body.

- *Unlocks the Elusive G-Spot* - In tantra, it is referred to as the sacred spot, the woman's most mysterious erogenous zone, which also happens to be the most potent. The G-spot is located approximately two to three inches up along the front wall of her vagina. In tantric philosophy, a lover who practices these ancient secret techniques can discover the body's direct sexual energy through its chakras.

- *It Promotes Feelings of Empowerment* - Images of perfection perpetuated by the media have made it easy for women to forget that they are beautiful just the way that they are. Tantric sex seeks to change that by helping women feel empowered by using their bodies to celebrate their desires. Women in tantric sex are treated with and given the respect and honor that they deserve. Their partners treat them with love and desire, worshipping their bodies like a goddess. This is beneficial for a woman's confidence and self-esteem.

- *It Promotes Healing* - Women, in general, are a lot more emotional than men. They wear their hearts on their sleeves, and past hurts, painful wounds or traumatic experiences have a way of leaving behind a scar that never really fades away. Tantra opens the door for a woman to heal from within, rooted in the teachings that call for a woman to be loved, honored, and respected not just in sex but in life too.

As for men, tantric sex is the better sex for the following reasons:

- *It Encourages Men to Understand Their Bodies Better* - Through tantra, men develop a greater understanding of their sexual energy and their bodies' response to pleasure. A lot of men do not pay enough attention to their bodies and their bodies' needs. With the focus so heavily concentrated on ejaculation, not enough attention is given towards what makes them feel good. Tantra's practices will change all of that through mindfulness. This, in turn, encourages better communicative skills while in bed with their partner and can help derive more pleasure when they can translate what they need.

- *Sex Becomes More Than Just What Porn Promotes* - Tantric sex teaches both men and women that the act of sex is more than just two people having intercourse. That sex is something to be treated as a sacred act, something which has deep meaning and lasting effects, even long after the sex part is over. From a very early age, men and boys are conditioned away from prolonged pleasure. They are also led to believe that their sexuality is to be reserved and at times, emotionless. This is exasperated by pornography that puts a false emphasis on ejaculation as the highest peak of pleasure and the primary goal. It is through tantric sex that men are awakened to the realization that sex should be treated with respect, cherished, and loved. It is one of the many reasons why it is so effective at deepening the bond between two people.

- *Achieving Multiple Orgasms* - It's no secret that most (if not all men) long to last longer and achieve multiple orgasms. A man can have whole-body, multiple orgasms, and can last for several minutes when tantric sex is involved. Part of tantra's teachings involve semen retention practices and learning how to transfer that ejaculation intensity into orgasmic energy; a man can have just as many orgasms as a woman. Semen is the life-force of a man; it must be kept in the body for a man to maintain his health. The act of ejaculation greatly reduces the life-force running through a male organism and is immediately followed by a drop in energy, creating a depressive nature. When semen is retained in the body, it directly supports the brain and central nervous system. It improves function, reinstating energy and confidence, and eventually leads to multiple orgasms for the men too.

- *Minimizes the Risk of Depression* - Men and women are both susceptible to depression. Especially with the pressures we face today. Tantra is one approach to minimizing the risk of depression because it encourages the elimination of negative energy and infuses both the mind and body with positive ones. The flow of energy movement and a heightened state of pleasure and bliss expels negative energy from the body

Mind-Blowing Techniques of Tantric Sex

There are two types of experiences that can be carried out by regular practitioners of tantric sex. Likewise, these are ideal for those who are already accustomed to performing the maithuna. Therefore, they are able to put charges into play with extraordinary energy. These are rituals dedicated to the Gods. Such practices are known in the West as "group sex."

In the first case, the energy load put into play is truly exceptional since in the ceremonies that are detailed here also summons the explicit invocation of one or more divinities– although all forms of maithuna are a way that a man and a woman summon their inner gods.

In the second case, during collective miathunas it's essential to bear in mind that they are not simply orgies as we might understand in the West. They are, though, energetic and spiritual ceremonies that utilizes sex as a path toward transcendence and enlightenment.

Shiva Shakty Ritual

- This ceremony aims to unify the consciousness, the connection to what's happening in this precise moment with eternity. Furthermore, it helps to overcome the boundaries of ego, time and space to access a higher plane.

- Bathe before starting the rite. The bath must be taken individually so that physical contact happens only during the beginning of the actual ritual.

- The man must wear yellow clothes preferably and, thus, representing the day, the sun and the masculine energy. The woman should be in black to symbolize the night, the moon, and the feminine energy.

- It is preferable that the room for the ceremony has a floor covered with carpets, cushions, and pillows. Furthermore, it must allow freedom of movement. It is also quite essential that there is a proper musical background. In addition, all inspiring decorations are welcome such as flowers, candles, incense, etc.

- Only once you've completed all of what was described before, create a circle in the room. This can be done either in a mental or physical way–through flower petals, a rope, or drawing the circle with chalk.

- Women and men stand in the center of the circle. Afterward, the women will place the palms of their hands on the middle of the chest and, looking at his partner in the eyes, he will recite: "I am the power of the feminine and the principle of life. I am Shakty. I am the girl, the woman, the companion, the mother, the wise, the magician, and the old woman. I receive you, Shiva, Man, God."

- In the same position, the man will say: "I am Shiva, power of the masculine, the light and spiritual impulse. I am the boy, the man, the partner, the father, the wise, the magician, and the patriarch. I receive you, Shakty, woman, Goddess."

- Then, both will say at the same time: "I offer you my dance." Afterward, you will begin to move your body freely within the circle. Be sure to always breathe slowly and deeply, in such a way that allows the dance to mobilize the energy within your bodies.

- As the body heat increases, you can start taking off your clothes–being careful that this always happens within the circle. In this way, you're offering your nudity to your partner in a physical and emotional sense.

- Continue dancing naked without touching each other for about 15 minutes and then sit face to face.

  Keep your back straight and your legs crossed. Stare into each other's eyes with love and devotion.

- Hold hands. Approximate your noses without touching each other and inhale the air that the other exhales, for not less than 15 minutes. This will allow the aura to be energetically fed back after the fatigue, which might have been caused due to dancing.

- At the end of the breathing stage, you'll begin to play throughout your bodies. Leave the genital until the very end.

- After several minutes of caresses, feel how the Kundalini energy has been already activated. The man will sit on the floor and the woman will climb on him so as to be penetrated.

- In this position, you'll perform smooth and delicate movements. It's crucial that you pay proper attention on breathing, making it as deep and as conscious as possible. It is important to keep in mind that this isn't just another sexual encounter. This is a special ritual. Due to that reason, the slower and deep breathing you perform, the chances decrease for the man to ejaculate before the woman reaches an orgasm. Furthermore, you'll both feel an ascension of energy.

- You and your partner will be able to mentally visualize Kundalini energy like a snake that unfolds through the ritual. In this way, the chakras are stimulated deeply.

- Once both of you've reached an orgasmic state, you'll stop on a smooth fashion until the ritual is over.

Kali Goddess Ritual

Kali is the passionate sexual initiator and the goddess who owns a supreme creative and destructive power. She does not know fear and is the one who transforms consciousness. The following ritual allows you to connect with anyone. What is more, the Kali Goddess Ritual helps to break the boundaries of the ego. Therefore, you'll be able to access a higher level of consciousness due to sensuality.

- During onenight, undress and draw a ritual circle (with petals, chalk, etc.) and start the ceremony by proclaiming the following sentence: "Kali, female spirit full of courage and passion, initiator Goddess of mysteries, bridge that unites the mundane and the transcendent, divinity capable of granting liberation through sex and wisdom: hold me in your arms. And with it, destroy my weaknesses and temper my spirit. Undress me from the inside so that I can see the light."

- Begin to dance erotically while feeling the atmosphere of the moment. At this point, you should attempt to connect through the movements with the energy of the Kali goddess. Visualize her as a beautiful woman with long black hair, four arms, and a beautifully curved body. She has very intense eyes and a long tongue which is held out and evoking the fire of sexual passion.

- At the middle of the dance, start repeating the mantra of Kali (Om kang kalika namah) for a minimum of 15 minutes. This was her presence and energy of Kali become more powerful and palpable.

- When you've considered that they you've recited the mantra enough times, move to a more meditative space. The man will close his eyes and visualize the mandala (mystical diagram) corresponding to the honored goddess, which are a series of five equilateral triangles inserted one inside the other and placed on a lotus flower with eight petals. At the center of it all, there's a small point that symbolizes the stability of consciousness.

- Once connected internally with Kali's mandala, the woman will support her body on her buttocks and will take the tip of her feet with each hand. She'll then lift them until he is in balance. The man will meditate on her naked yoni and will kiss her and drink from her energetic fluids.

- The man will lie on his back, relaxing his body, and the woman, incarnating Kali will stand on top of him.

- The male will touch the erogenous zones of his partner's body.

- When they feel that desire is truly powerful, the woman will stick out her tongue as much as possible. Afterward, she'll introduce the lingam in her wet yoni. Then they will perform the maithuna. Stay in this position so as to allow the undulating movements of the body of the goddess Kali embodied in the woman.

- With the sexual organs together, men and women will repeat the mantra of Kali again every time they're exhalating. This will allow you to completely loosen up your individual egos and reach a sexual and spiritual climax. After that, you too then stay in a state of complete silence, bliss and meditative ecstasy.

- Finish the ritual by thanking Kali.

Collective Maithunas

Part of the tantric tradition argues that emotions can be exalted if there's the presence of a third party or somebody else participating in a form of collective sexual rituals. Tantra affirms that sex between three or more people if it's practiced for a spiritual sake. The most common forms of collective maithunas are the sexual encounters that are performed with two women and one man. The woman has an eminently receptive nature. Furthermore, because among most of them there is a feeling of brotherly solidarity, eroticism and sensuality, which consequently generates attraction and unity. These collective sex encounters are called by Tantra "Secret Games." Its importance is such that it was a common practice among Indian emperors and kings.

The sacred tantric book of Chandamaharosana describes group sex in the following way: "A woman from the moon is enjoyed by another one similar to her. The third person differs from the other two and must balance her strength. When enjoyed together, they all free themselves from decay and of death. He stimulates them both. They excite each other and they combine with him. The two moons are always full of nectar and the sun burns without being consumed." For the purpose of unity for three to occur, self-interest and strong emotions should disappear. Otherwise, these experiences would become something mundane, far from the tantric goal of transcendence.

Another sexual practice of a collective nature is the so-called Ritual of the Five Senses. This ritual consists of the union of a man with five different women, in which each of them represents a different sense. This way, the five senses are stimulated to obtain spiritual liberation.

Chakra Puja Ritual

Chakra Puja means "circular cult" and is performed with eight couples (man-woman). Each of them makes up a circle and have their own encounters. The ritual consists of stopping before reaching an orgasm. Afterward, the couple begins to have sex and stops before the climax. They do the same, and they go on. This way, a very powerful accumulation of energy is created. This particular ritual allows participants to reach a state of ecstasy besides erotic enjoyment.

Yoguini Chakra Ritual

In the past, this rite was practiced by tantric monarchs to procreate enlighten children. This ritual is practiced between a man and an odd number of women–e.g. three, five, or seven of them. The man and his partner are placed in the center while surrounded by the remaining women. Alternatively, each woman will have a short encounter with the man. The man would not spread his semen to the other women. He'd absorb the women's energy to finally grant it to his partner.

Bhairavi Chakra Ritual

A woman stands naked in the center of a circle, representing the goddess Kali. The couples participating in the rite offer her flowers, fruits, and drinks. After doing so, they make up a circle and then they start performing the maithuna.

Group Sex in the Kama Sutra

According to the Kama Sutra, when a man enjoys two women at the same time, he should love them equally. When a man performs maithuna at the same time with several women, this union is called "the pack of cows." There are several types of unions and some of them are as following:

- The water union (which is also known as the elephant union) is a ritual only takes places in the water.

- The union of the pack of goats or the union of the pack of hinds, is called due to its similarity to the movements of this animal.

- In some cases, several young men practice maithuna with a woman who may be the partner of one of them. One holds her, while the other enjoys her. A third man over her mouth, a fourth caresses her navel. Each man alternates in each position.

Sexual Arousal and Excitement

To achieve ultimate arousal, foreplay must be done properly. Tantric sex involves meditation and connecting the energy from the sexual organs to your heart, so to speak. You can accomplish your goal using the following steps.

Meditate With Your Partner

Meditation must be a vital part of your daily schedule, even if you don't make love. Meditating daily or regularly will relax your nerves and alleviate stress. You may not know it, but one main reason for an inability to enjoy sex and achieve orgasm is stress and depression.

Find a peaceful and quiet corner and meditate with your partner. Choose a place where no one can disturb you. Make sure the place is comfortable, clean and safe. Do breathing exercises while facing each other. Feel the energy between your bodies and allow this energy to flow to your partner.

- Inhale deeply with your nose
- Wait for 6 seconds
- Exhale forcefully with your nose and mouth

While inhaling deeply, mentally instruct each muscle of your body to relax; starting from your toes to the top of your head. Do this again in reverse – from the top of your head down to your toes.

Tantric meditation is similar to mindfulness meditation. They have the same goal: to be aware of things around you in a relaxed state. Use this to know more about yourself so you can succeed in your goals.

Tantra meditation has three main components. These are Mantra, Meditation and full body cosmic orgasms.

Other practitioners use Yoga Nidra meditation, which is a deeper form of meditation. However, you don't have to go into that as a beginner.

Visualize the energy of a supreme being from the cosmos coursing through your body, providing you with positive energy. Some of those who are deep into Tantra imagine themselves to be gods.

You can also use mantras to enhance your meditation. The important thing is to create awareness while relaxing your mind, body and spirit.

Be Positive

Optimism is always one of your tickets to success in anything you do. Learning how to view events with a positive mentality will help your overcome your mistakes and start over again.

If you have a positive outlook, half of the battle is already won. Look forward to the happening as a chance to strengthen your relationship and achieve your long-time sexual fantasy of having multiple orgasms.

Take a Shower

Personal hygiene is part of good sex, so take your shower first. This is a step that may be omitted by others. You can start foreplay while showering, or you can shower separately and then proceed to the bedroom naked.

If you decide to shower together, slowly lather each other while massaging and fondling your body parts. Don't stay long in the shower. And no! You can't consummate the act while in the shower! Continue with your foreplay once you are in the bedroom.

Eliminate Lust from Your System

Tantric sex has never been about lust, so first get that out of your system. Being so pumped up by lust at the start is detrimental to Tantric sex. With that thought in mind, start or continue with foreplay. Control your passion. Tantric sex is not about "quickies." Learn how to control your reactions. That's why it is critical that you learn how to meditate before the actual sexual intercourse. Meditating will help you overcome your emotions and lust.

Pray and Play Together For Your Foreplay

This is best done on a clean floor, with a soft mat and some pillows. Offer a short prayer together to your spiritual being. Close your eyes and visualize the spiritual connection coming from your partner. You may listen to soft, beautiful music to help you get in the mood. Choose the music that calms and de-stresses you.

After the prayer, hold hands and look at each other. Admire what you see. Relish the time to be able to gaze at your loved one. When you feel that the energy is starting to build again, stand up and dance. Dance a slow dance while savoring the warmth that courses through your bodies. Stay close to each other. Move your bodies together and against each other. Bask in the music and the joy of being together.

Afterwards, the woman can sit on the lap of the man. If you're the man, position yourself so that you are facing each other and your partner's buttocks are resting gently atop your lap. Harmonize your breathing by alternating inhalation and exhalation; when she inhales, you exhale; when she exhales, you inhale. Gaze into each other's eyes again and focus on the emotions generated by your proximity to one another. Visualize the energy flowing back and forth between your two bodies.

Do this until you can feel its impact? There should be a palpable energy throbbing and pulsating within and around your bodies.

Tantric Foreplay through Massage to Remove Energy Blocks

Massage each other's bodies using clockwise and counterclockwise hand massages. Use your thumbs as you massage every inch of your partner's body. Imagine the energy flowing back and forth between your fingers and their body.

Feel each pulsating, throbbing body part, where the energy is freely flowing. You can detect the energy blocks when the area doesn't pulsate, or is cold or painful. Gently massage this block until it becomes warm. Sense the energy from your fingers successfully removing the energy block. Inch by inch, massage each other's bodies in slow, unhurried movements. Enjoy the blissful sensations evoked from these areas of contact.

When you come to the genitals, be tender. These are your partner's most sensitive parts. Take it slow, and delight in each touch. Feel the pulsation of each other's heart and allow the energy to flow between you. The woman's breasts must now be tingling with the energy, sensuously pulsating. The male's manhood may now be tumescent by the free-flowing energy coming from his partner. You can close your eyes to savor the ecstatic sensation. Remember to breathe slowly and relax.

Consummate the Sexual Act Using Tantric Intercourse

You're now ready for penetration. If you have performed the massage correctly, you can feel the vibrant energy pulsating in your bodies. Think of the consummation of the act as the union of the male and female energies. The male joins the woman at the groin, while the woman presses her breasts against the chest of the man to unite their sexual energies at the heart chakra.

Again, take it slow! Avoid thrusting like an animal in heat. Tantric sex is about slow movements and basking in the incredible sensations that each movement elicits. The man should penetrate slowly inside his partner, savoring each thrust. Feel the energy sensations going up and down your spine. Remember to relax and be totally conscious of each other's bodies. You should experience full body orgasms during this period.

When you reach orgasm, feel it flowing to your brain and into your heart. Don't limit the sensation by focusing on your groin and pelvic area. Let it reach your mind and spirit. Allow yourself to soar to the high heavens.

Proceed to Tantra Samadhi

This is the period after both of you have reached orgasm. You now lay still and relax. Hold hands and go into a deep state of relaxation. This will further intensify your orgasm. It's only when you're relaxed that your spirituality can merge with your physical body and the cosmic world around you. You should feel a cosmic bliss that transcends your physical bodies.

Proceed to Tantric Transformation

Your orgasm can never transcend the physical if you don't tap into your Tantra and complete the merging of your body, brain, heart and soul. When the body and soul unify, the transcendental orgasm occurs, and this cannot be equaled by the physical orgasm that most people are so excited about. This is also called the heart orgasm, or energy orgasm. Together with your practice of Tantric sex, your life will take a turn for the better. You'll learn how to tap into the energy of your inner self and the cosmos to create energy fields of successes around you.

Tantric Massage, Meditation And Yoga

Tantric Massage

Massage is defined as a succession of strokes performed to promote muscular relaxation. However, tantric massage is more than that. The tantric touch stimulates, nurtures, and heals the body, the mind, the emotions, and the spirit.

When done on its own, tantric massage can be an erotic experience. It can also turn into a therapeutic journey. When done prior to sex, tantric massage is a means of prolonging and building pleasure. When used as foreplay, the tantric touch relaxes your mind and your body so it becomes more receptive to your partner's gifts. It enables your sexual arousal to mount before it reaches its pinnacle. This way, your orgasms can become longer and more intense.

Tantric sex is safe and healthy lovemaking. In the early dating phase, some couples may feel pressured to engage in intercourse before they're emotionally attached or psychologically prepared. Using tantric massage as a pleasurable alternative for intercourse relieves them of this pressure. Tantric massage can be a fun and sexy way of getting to know each other deeper so that you'll have ample time to emotionally connect with each other. This way, once you finally decide to have sex, it becomes more meaningful and more satisfying.

Benefits of Tantric Massage

The busy and hectic life that we lead these days affects both men and women, and it causes several physical, emotional, and even sexual disorders. Stress doesn't discriminate, and it could trouble a person belonging to any age group, sex, or age. People need some relief if they want to enjoy their life to the fullest and they also have to replenish their strength to keep up with their hectic lifestyle. Massage can help in providing the much-needed comfort and help you relax.

Among all the different types of massages that exist, tantric massage is gaining popularity. The main aim of a tantric massage is to provide you with a sensual experience that will also help in improving your health. Even though it is erotic, it helps the whole body to relax and has got several benefits.

Stress Buster

Tantric massage can help you clear your mind, make your body feel light, and help you relax. You can let go of all the tension and stress. Therefore, a session of tantric massage is recommended whenever you feel stressed. Stress is something that is capable of making you feel miserable, and if it isn't handled properly, it can cause several health problems as well.

Sex education

In many cultures around the world, sex education isn't adequate, and this leaves both the genders unprepared for any sexual interaction or even sensuality. A tantric massage is the best way in which you can learn about your body. It provides you with a serial interaction that will help you to understand how your body works. It provides you with an insight into how your body works and the different parts that will make you feel different sensations. When you do interact with your partner, it will be helpful to know beforehand itself what excites and pleases you both.

Premature ejaculation

Premature ejaculation usually tends to occur due to the pressure of performance. In most of the societies and cultures, men are considered to be the "doers," and this does put an added pressure of performance of them and causes them to ejaculate prematurely. Tantric massage helps in taking this pressure off them and lets them just enjoy the sexual act. When there isn't an expectation of them to perform well and without any specific goal in mind, men can perform well sexually. This will help in rectifying the problem of premature ejaculation. Tantric massage will help in teaching you to enjoy the moment, and during intercourse, it would also improve a man's ability to hold off his climax for a while longer. It is all about drawing out the pleasure to make the experience more intense.

Orgasm in older men

As the time passes by, and while the body starts aging, the hormone levels in the body tend to decline and because of this older man feel little or even no sexual arousal and this means that they aren't capable of reaching an orgasm. Tantric massage can be beneficial for older men. This sensual massage helps in stimulating their senses and also helps in the production of the sex hormones and thereby helping them deal with problems like erectile dysfunction and the lack of achieving an orgasm.

Women and sex

In most of the cases, women don't enjoy intercourse. This could be caused due to various reasons ranging from their lover's inability to please them or even their lack of knowledge about their body. Women are sensual creatures, and it takes them a while longer to achieve an orgasm. Most might not even be aware of their bodies or what they like and dislike. Tantric massage will help them in understanding their bodies and their needs better. It will help them in deriving greater pleasure and even sensuality during any form of sexual activity.

Tantric massage helps in awakening your senses. It is sensual, we tend to perceive the world around us through our senses, and the awakening of the senses sharpens this perception of ours. Tantric massage is a therapeutic massage that has various health benefits. It can help in relieving body pains and aches, stimulating your immune system, and increasing your fertility as well. Many women can't orgasm, and tantric massage helps in integrating your mind and body thereby facilitating their ability to reach an orgasm. Tantric massage tends to be empowering on various levels regardless of the characteristics of an individual. Tantric massage also helps in providing the greatest form of relaxation and pleasure for your mind, body, and soul without having to reciprocate. Tantric massage involves the massaging of all the parts of the body. Having one's genitals massaged is quite a fulfilling experience. It also helps in creating a conscious connection between all the areas of a person's life. A massage without any expectations is quite a liberating experience. Tantric massage helps in letting go of the illusion of separation that exists and remedies this divide that exists in every individual's life. It can also pave the way for a full-body orgasm.

Tantric Meditation

Many people imagine meditation as complete stillness of the mind. They imagine sitting cross-legged or in the lotus position and chanting "Ohm."
However, there are many ways to meditate. In fact, nearly any activity can be turned into a meditative act. The secret is in not trying to block all thoughts from entering, but rather to welcome them and let them pass. Do not hold on to any one particular thought. You are in your meditative state to relax, not to fight incoming thoughts. The important thing is to avoid obsessing over problems or worrying about negative thoughts.
Start by finding a comfortable place without any distractions. In other words, no telephone, television, children, or chores. (This can be a challenge, but it will be worth the trouble.) Make yourself comfortable. Begin by taking deep breaths, all the way into your abdomen. Feel how your stomach expands as you inhale. Now exhale. Let all of the air out. Empty your lungs completely.
There are several relaxation techniques you can use as well. Try tightening and relaxing each part of your body one at a time, from your feet to your forehead. You can imagine inhaling light and exhaling all negativities.

Traditional Tantric Meditation Technique

Tantric meditation takes this basic meditation technique and expands upon it. Through practice, the Tantric can enter into a state of complete relaxation. From there, Tantra teaches that she or he will become conscious of the life force within. The Tantric will direct this energy from the base of the spine, up to the neck, and finally to the forehead. Tantric can then, with experience, direct that life energy out from the forehead and form a body of energy before him or her. The body of energy will become denser and expand until reaching human size.

Tantric Yoga

Tantric yoga helps in improving the nature of one's relationship and cherishing and furthermore for imparting delicate exercise to accomplices. As it were it is an easy to-execute yoga routine for sex accomplices to build the progression of sex yielding energy. It additionally helps in a standard practice for making your body resistible, with a decent body, personality and soul both inside and outside the room.

Straightforward Yoga movements

This segment will enable you to get familiar with a couple of fundamental yoga represents that you can perform to improve your general wellbeing and stamina. In the following segment, you will learn about the diverse tantric activities that you can, and your accomplice can perform together. This will help in expanding your closeness and solace level with each other.

The Head lift

Ensure that you are standing up straight for this. At that point tilt your head upward what's more, tilt it in such a way, that string from the sky was pulling it upwards. Keep your mouth shut, and you should breathe in through your nose. When you are breathing in, ensure that you are moving your shoulder bones in reverse so that it would appear that they are attempting to contact one another. It should feel like your feet are fixed to the ground. Loosen up your position and afterward rehash this procedure.

The Cobra postures

You can rest on the floor or a yoga tangle. Presently stretch out your body to make sure that your stomach is contacting the floor. At that point place your hands under your bears with the goal that your elbows are set at the back. Lift your chest off the floor also, tilt your head with the goal that it would seem that a bend. Ensure that you are looking upwards. This posture should like a cobra that is going to strike. Loosen up your position and after that recurrent this procedure.

The Cat postures

When you are finished with the Cobra present, you should delicately bring down your head furthermore, gradually ascend on your knees. This should appear as though you are squatting, so stretch your spine the other way than what you did in the Cobra present.

The Resting postures

When you have completed the Cat present, you should expect the Cobra present. Stretch your arms outwards. Take in profoundly and unreservedly. Ensure that your temple is laying on the ground and that your chest is contacting your knees.

Tantric exercises

If you need to add some use to your routine with regards to Tantric sex, at that point you can start rehearsing a couple of activities and breathing procedures that will help you in making your sexual experience far and away superior. These activities, just as relaxing systems, are most appropriate when finished with your accomplice, yet they should be possible on your own also. These activities and breathing systems have been referenced in this segment.

Shoulder stand

Shoulder stands are useful for ladies for accepting the different Tantric stances effortlessly, yet on the other hand men can rehearse them also. For playing out a basic shoulder represent, the individual should rests level on a tangle or even the floor with his/her legs extended straight and their hands resting close by. The individual will at that point need to lift the legs at a 90-degree edge with the goal that their upper middle stays stuck to the floor. Their legs ought to be lifted somewhat higher than their lower back, and their hands ought to be put on their back for supporting this pose. Rehearsing this strategy will help in building up the truly necessary adaptability for accepting different Tantric sex positions.

Boat posture

This posture is by and by supportive for ladies. The individual playing out this posture ought to sit with a straight back, and their legs ought to be loosened up. At that point the individual should lift their legs at a 45-degree point and after that stretch their hands outwards with the goal that their fingers are pointing towards their feet. Attempt and keep up this posture for three minutes and after that unwind. Rehash this posture multiple times.

Three-legged pooch posture

This posture is useful for extending the hamstring muscles, and these are very regularly utilized in Tantric sex. For playing out this represent, the individual must lie down on their stomach on a tangle while their hands are set on their sides. Your palms ought to be set alongside the chest and bolster your feet with your toes. Lift your body in such a way, that your toes bolster your body weight. This position ought to appear as though your body is making a triangle, with the floor framing the base of the triangle. The correct leg should then be gradually lifted upwards. Lift your leg to the extent your body would allow. At that point come back to nonpartisan position and rehash the equivalent with the other leg.

Extension posture

This is a represent that is appropriate for both the genders. For playing out this procedure, you should rest on your back and after that twist your legs in such a way so your knees are pointing upwards. Your feet ought to be set near your bum. The lower middle ought to be lifted, and your hands should lie on either side of your body for offering help. Rehash these multiple times.

Kegels

This posture will help ladies in reinforcing their pelvic muscles. This aides in fixing the hold of the pelvic muscles and for making the vaginal part appear to be more tightly, in this way making it an undeniably all the more invigorating knowledge for both parties. For playing out this activity, the lady should focus on the vaginal muscles and draw them in and discharge. The suction can be clutched for as long as could reasonably be expected and afterward discharged. This activity should be possible anyplace and at any purpose of time. It likewise enables muscle to control extensively.

Kapalbhatti

This is a simple breathing procedure, and the man can play out this privilege previously his orgasm. This can likewise be played out each morning for better outcomes. For playing out this procedure, you will essentially need to take a few short and sharp breaths. It is ideal to do this while sitting upstanding with your legs jumbled. The focal point of this activity is more on the exhalation of air than inward breath. The mouth ought to be shut while breathing out and this ought to make an uproarious sound while letting the fresh up. Play out this in sets of 3.

Pranayama

This is another activity that can be performed by both the genders and it helps in helping and controlling your breathing during Tantric sex. For playing out this strategy, the individual can sit upstanding in the lotus posture and spot the correct thumb on their correct nostril and point a finger at the focal point of your temple. Breath in through your left nostril, hold the breath for a couple of moments and after that discharge it through your correct nostril. While doing this, the correct nostril ought to be liberated, and the left nostril ought to be squeezed up. Rehash these multiple times. This can help the energy levels to increment and furthermore helps mindfulness.

The objective of this activity is to set up the body, brain and soul for more profound closeness.

Benefits of Practicing Tantra

In addition to the general benefits mentioned above, tantra yoga is known to benefit by helping people deal with the following conditions by taking advantage of increased energy levels in the body:

- Stiffness in the body

- Stress and anxiety

- General fatigue

- Shoulder and back problems

While enlightenment may not happen overnight by Tantra practices (as it is not some kind of flashy miracle operation), sustained efforts at getting the right techniques and performing them patiently will go a long way in improving your spiritual and physical well-being. Of course, a healthy body is a prerequisite to achieve awakened states of consciousness and this theory is valid for all the systems present in this world. Healthy eating combined with a healthy lifestyle is critical to ensuring the successful outcome of any holistic healing system.

Tantric Sex Position

The Sidewinder

This position is enlivened from the yoga position of a similar name, and this procedure takes into account deep entrance. It likewise accommodates the couple to keep in touch. For playing out this method, the lady should rests on her side and supports the heaviness of her chest area with the assistance of her hands. She should lift one of her legs and place it on her darling's shoulder while the other leg is lying on the bed. A variety of this equivalent position is that then again the man can rests behind the lady and enter his partner from behind.

The Yab Yum

The Yab Yum position is viewed as probably the best situation for having tantric sex. It is a genuinely simple situation to perform, and it takes into consideration synchronous climaxes. This position helps in animating quite a few places. Likewise, the man's hands happen to be free right now, he can touch his darling's body however he sees fit, since the couple would confront one another, it takes into consideration enthusiastic kisses also. The man should sit leg over leg on the bed or some other agreeable surface and hold his back straight. The lady should straddle him and fold her legs over his lower back.

The Latch

This posture permits the man to get a decent see his sweetheart's face and the other way around. This is an extremely attractive posture and aides in pleasuring both the partners. For playing out this procedure, the lady should be situated on a high stage like a table or even the kitchen counter. She will then need to recline and adjust her upper middle and her head with the assistance of her hands by inclining onto her elbows. The man should remain between her separated legs and enter her. This is one represent that doesn't need to be limited to the room and is ideal for an off the cuff cavort.

The Butterfly

This method is accepted to allow both the partners to achieve a significant level of rapture and takes into consideration deep entrance. For playing out this system, the young lady should rests on the table so that her butt lies at the edge of the table and the man should help lift her lower back marginally off the table and afterward place both her legs over his shoulders. Her vagina would be free for him to infiltrate while remaining in the middle of her legs. Since her legs are shut together, this fixes the vaginal waterway and gives a tight fit. The man should enter her while her butt is in midair.

The Double Decker

This is an amazingly suggestive posture and will help in accomplishing a climax no problem at all. The man will likewise be given a decent perspective on all the activity that is going on down there, and his hands will likewise have unlimited access to lay with his sweetheart's butt. This position is very enabling for ladies since they have all the control here. For playing out this system, the man should sit on the bed while his legs are collapsed under his body. The lady will then need to confront away from him and place her feet one either side of her darling while her feet are set level superficially to give her some help. When she has brought down herself onto his erect penis, then she will just need to begin moving advances and in reverse or can even decide on a here and there movement. The man should basically kick back and have fun.

Skiff

This position is a slight adjustment of the lady on top position. Right now, bodies should be situated so that both the partners will find a good pace great take a gander at one another's face while occupied with the demonstration. For playing out this, the man should sit down on a seat that can marginally twist in reverse. The lady will then need to put herself on his lap and afterward place her legs on either side of the seat. The young lady should fire an allover development without anyone else, or her partner can help her by setting his hand under her bum and helping her move in an upwards and downwards way.

The Mermaid

This is a somewhat fluctuated adaptation of the butterfly, and it takes into consideration a more solace and better hold. Right now, man can play with his darling's feet. Remember that feet are viewed as one of the most touchy and erogenous pieces of a lady's body. For playing out this method, the lady should expect a similar situation as she did in the butterfly, however her butt ought to be propped with the assistance of a pad. Her legs should loosen up and ought to be at a 90-degree edge. The man should stand near the table and infiltrate her.

Tsunami

This posture is very agreeable, and it is a sensual treat. This will knock your socks off. This posture is a slight alteration of the exemplary minister style. Right now, lady should expect the job that a man as a rule does in the teacher style. For playing out this, the man should rests level on his back, and his arms should be put close by. The lady should lie over him, and the man should embed his penis into her vagina. The lady should totally loosen up her legs with the goal that they are resting on his. Her palms ought to be put on his lower arm for giving her some help. The lady will then need to begin moving her pelvis in an upward and descending development.

Lap Dance

This is a great posture for a man to encounter his darling's body in the entirety of its magnificence. His hands will be allowed to meander around her body, and he can do what he needs. The lady will face away from him as she would have, had she been giving him a lap move. For playing out this represent, the man should sit down on a seat, and his back should be kept straight. The lady will then sit on his lap and parity herself by setting her hands on his upper thighs or even his stomach. She will then need to lift herself gradually and place the backs of her calves and brings down herself onto his penis.

Pretzel

This is another represent that is satisfying to take a gander at and even simple to expect. This will cause the couple to feel incredibly attractive. For playing out this procedure, the couple should stop before one another. The man should move advances, and the lady will fold her arms over him. The lady will then lift herself up and place her left leg by her darling's correct foot; her foot will confront downwards. The man will then need to put his left leg close to her correct foot. When taken a gander at a couple occupied with this posture, they look like a pretzel, an extremely provocative and mouth-watering pretzel.

The Spread

This is an essential and an amazingly hot position. This permits the lady to get incredible delight since it lets her stroke her sweetheart and permits him the entrance to joy her. For playing out this system, the lady should sit at the very edge of the couch or even the bed and spread her legs separated. The man will then need to remain in the middle of her legs and infiltrate her. She can draw nearer to him and kiss him while his hands have the entrance to her full body.

The Entwine

This posture looks intense and about difficult to copy, however then it very well may be pleasurable if it's done appropriately. This posture is tastefully engaging. For playing out this strategy, the couple should sit near one another and face each other. The man should put his legs on either side of his partner. The lady will then need to lift both of her legs and place them on either side of her sweetheart's sides, under his arms. The man's upper arms will secure the lady's legs, and the lady will then need to lift her upper arms and place them over his elbows. The man will then lift his legs and place them over her hands. This does sound very muddled, isn't that right? All the exertion that goes into it will merit your time and energy.

The G-force

This is maybe one of the most blazing tantric sex presents there is. This is the piece de opposition of all sex presents. The man has full oversight over his darling right now, both the people included will get extraordinary delight from this posture. For playing out this position, the lady should rests on her back on the bed, and the man must bow by her legs. He will then gradually lift her middle off the bed so she's offsetting herself with her head and her shoulders put on the bed. The man can either extend her legs at a 90-degree edge or infiltrate her, or he can likewise pull them separated and place her feet just beneath his chest and enter her.

The Waterfall

Right now, lady should put her hand on her sweetheart's penis and afterward let her fingertips brush his scrotum gradually and tenderly. It is a smart thought to use some ointment for making it progressively pleasurable. Her hands should be set on either side of his gonads, and afterward she should gradually slide her hands up till they arrive at the touchy tip of his penis. When this is done, the lady should give the man some time to chill off, and he will then need to respond the administration he got. The man needs to cup his sweetheart's vagina and touch all her delicate spots. He should slide his hands over her clitoris and her vaginal external lips.

The Snake

For this, the lady should gradually extend the pole of her sweetheart's penis with one of her hands and let the other hand follow little circles directly under the leader of the pole. This is like giving a slow and delicate hand work. Proceed with these movements a clockwise way and afterward once you arrive at the leader of the penis move to anticlockwise heading. Keep this up for whatever length of time that your sweetheart can suffer it.

Tantric Triangle of Touch

The lady should rests on her back and spread her legs somewhat and twist them at the knee. The man will then need to embed his list and center finger into her vagina and marginally twist them upwards till they make a come here development. This will give the ideal incitement to her G-Spot. This will make her groan in delight. While doing this, he should put the palm of his other hand on her lower midriff and apply a little delight. This consolidated incitement will rapidly push her off the edge.

The Teeter-Totter

There is nothing remotely guiltless about this specific teeter-totter. This is exceptionally suggestive. The lady should rests on her back on the bed, and her pelvis should be somewhat tilted upwards. A pad can be propped under her pelvis for doing as such. The man will then need to lift her feet and tenderly overlap them with the goal that her knees are laying on her bosoms and the bottoms of her feet are touching his chest. This position permits unhindered access to a lady's vagina, and the upward tilt will guarantee that he hits her G-Spot each time he pushes into her.

Tub Tangle

Get your man to lean back in a tub that is loaded up with water and the lady should straddle him while her back is confronting him. When his penis has entered her, he should sit up so you both are confronting one another. Then she should fold her legs over him, and he will do likewise with the goal that their elbows are under their partner's knees. Clutch each other as firmly as you can and start an influencing to and fro movement. This allows for some enthusiastic kissing.

Love Triangle

The lady should rests on her back on the floor or the bed and afterward she should lift her left advantage into the air. Her correct legs ought to be loosened up to her correct side, with the end goal that both her legs are lying opposite to one another. She will then need to move her correct hand and catch her correct knee and form a triangle on the bed with the use of her correct leg and her correct hand. The man should hunch a little and enter her while holding her knee. This position would give the man better pelvic control and furthermore the chance of touching from multiple points of view as you would need to.

Presently and Zen

This posture can be used for giving a snapshot of relief from the approaching climax. Tantric sex isn't tied in with discovering speedy discharge; it is tied in with enjoying the experience. What better approach to do as such, than to control yourself directly before arriving at the final turning point. When you feel that it is possible that you or your partner is near climaxing, enjoy a couple of moments and reprieve liberated from the position that you both are in. Slow pushing is passable, however if you feel that, you are going to climax, then pause for a minute, delay, maybe appreciate a tad of kissing and touching before proceeding with where you had given up. This position gives the genuinely necessary closeness during the sex to make the entire experience additionally adoring and healthy.

Torrid Tug-of-War

The lady should sit leg over leg on the floor or some other agreeable surface and afterward gradually sink onto his erect penis and fold her legs over his back. This position will permit the couple to confront one another and this implies you can grasp each other's elbows for offering some help and incline toward the bearing endlessly from your partner. If you both happen to be adaptable, then one partner can tilt their heads back and lean in reverse, away from the other partner. This position will take into account the arrangement of your bodies, and it will cause you to associate with your partner.

X Marks the Spot

Right now, lady must rests on the bed or some other delicate surface of decision with her head propped on a pad. She should bring her knees up to her chest and fold her legs at her lower legs. The man will then need to stoop before her and gradually lean in some time pulling her hips towards his crotch. She should keep her thighs squeezed together while he begins pushing into her.

Arc de Triomphe

This is a serious hot posture. The man should sit down on the bed with his legs extended before him. His sweetheart should slither up to him and afterward straddle his erect part. When you both are agreeable right now, should curve her back as much as she can. Being adaptable will prove to be useful right now. The man should lean forward and begin pushing into her. Ladies should prepare themselves for the invasion of development by clutching their lower legs. The man will find a workable pace all-encompassing perspective on his sweetheart's body and devour it. If the man wishes along these lines, he can lean down and kiss her chest too.

Head Game

Right now, lady should rests on the ground or some other level surface while her face is confronting upwards. Her hands should support her lower body; she will then need to lift her advantages, and her back too with the goal that they are lying opposite to the ground. She can support her pressure by propping up her arms against her lower back. While she is clutching her lower legs, the man should stop before her and bring his knees towards her shoulders. This is topsy-turvy activity, ensure that you are delicate with your darling and it very well may be very dubious to get it directly in the first go itself.

Supernova

This is a represent that essentially begins by appearing as though a standard cowgirl position. Rather than the lady mounting him the long way, she should mount him while lying opposite to him on the bed. When she detects her man moving toward a climax, she can tenderly crush on his middle and incline toward her knees and continue crawling forward towards the edge of the bed with the goal that his head and shoulders are hanging off the side of the bed. This position puts all the control with the lady, and she can ride her man, in any case, she satisfies. It is very engaging to the Goddess to see that she has the reigns right now. Tastefully, it is a serious sight for the man to view.

Love Seat

The man should rests on his back and prop his head with the assistance of a couple of cushions and spread his legs marginally. The lady should bring down herself onto his erect penis while confronting endlessly from him. It resembles the turnaround cowgirl position. She should put her feet between his legs on either side of the floor or the bed that he's lying on. Her right-hand should be put on the correct side of his hip and the left one on the left side. His hands are allowed to wander her body. Indeed, the inward goddess will be glad and will savor the control that has been put in her grasp.

Tantric Erotic Massage

Tantric massage is a path toward touch—the divine touch. It's slow, loving, artistic and sensuous. Unlike a typical hand job, tantric massage focuses on building sensual delight and releasing tension, with emphasis placed on healing the body and mind. When you know why you are touching, it becomes easier even for you to tailor your touch to your agenda. In this case, your intention is to heal, and not to arouse. The following expert tips should help any person out to try tantric massage.

Prior to performing your massage, you must first create an ambience of excitement—one of sensuality. One way of doing that is dimming the lights, or alternatively, go for candles.

Check to confirm that your room temperature is enabling, and not too hot or cold. Give the room some scent or simply settle for scented candles. In the background, you can also play some cool music, one that resonates well with your partner. You will also need some baby wipes, a towel, blindfold, and of course massage oil

Take Time to Connect

Prior to getting touchy, take a few minutes to connect first to yourself. You can do this by closing your eyes followed by some deep breath. When already in touch with yourself, connect with your lover by making contact with one another.

Use Quality Oils

Oil plays a key role in tantric massage, and you don't want to mess things up before you even start. Your oil should be 100% natural, scented and one with prolonged lubrication effect. You can use Rose oil, Sandalwood oil, Grape seed oil, or any other oil with the above qualities.

Other great tips include:

- Focus on all your body, including hair, eyelashes, lips, breath, and much more

- Perform the strokes sensuously and creatively

- Use sufficient amounts of the right natural oil

- Always give your lover some eye contact

- Enjoy the waves of internal pleasure with your lover

- Be adventurous, but always communicate with your lover to be sure of their comfort

- Make known your fantasies and sexual preferences

- Don't simply pour oil on your lover's body. Have the oil in your palm instead, and warm it a little bit before applying it to her body

- Always ask for her feedback

- Carry out the massage on your floor and not bed. The uneven nature of your mattress may result to extra back pain for your lover

Man Massaging a Woman

It is best referred to as male to female Tantra massage. It is very refreshing, energizing and invigorating. If you have a partner and you would like to give her this massage that combines sexual energy with traditional massage techniques, learn it!

Tantra massage is very important for women because it helps them awaken internal sexual goddesses in environments that are safe to nurture spiritual, physical and emotional satisfaction. For women, it is a special way of healing pain from separation, deficiency of love and even abuse using meditation, gentle pleasuring and visualization. Tantric massage further addresses experiences that turn a lady off, fading love in relationships, poor knowledge, trauma and pain. The main question that many ladies ask is whether their masseur should be a man or a woman. Here is what to expect in tantric massage from a man to a woman.

Between women and men, erotic tension is deeply ingrained in the complex dynamics of curiosity and sexual attractiveness is a turn on.

With a male masseur, a woman can explore herself fully to ensure she can handle her man while still being in control of herself. Men have sensitive hands by the way, which can be used to drive all the stress and fatigue out of the body of a woman.

Men masseurs give women greater pleasure because massage comes with the real experience of being with a man just like home. For couples on training, it will be easy to repeat for unending pleasure and reunion at home.

How far will a male masseur go?

The limits of any tantric massage session are set before commencement. This is important to guarantee clients of their safety.

If the masseur is your partner, lover or husband, they can go all the way, since this is a happy ending massage. If it is a professional masseur, set the boundaries in advance and know how far to go. However, there is nothing to prevent you from enjoying an explosive sexual ending as long as there is mutual consent.

When you are massaging her at home

Compression - This is where you use two hands, palms down to apply pressure on certain areas of the body. This causes the blood to flow to that area and the muscles relax in a big way. This massage technique is best performed on expansive areas of the body like the shoulders and the back.

The stroking technique – It is very easy to perform this one. You just need to use the whole of your palm, and give long strokes while at the same time applying gentle but firm pressure on the muscles. It is very rewarding and she will love you for it. You can use the long strokes on every area of her lovely body; say, you could even use it from the toes to the hips, from the neck to the buttocks and so on. Keep your fingers straight, even the thumb. She will love this.

Using the friction method – This is also a common method that you can use on a woman. It involves firm rubbing on the fingers and the palms against a part of the body. It does not need you to use oils, but then you should be a bit gentle with the skin of your lover. Experts say that this is an advanced technique, but you can perfect it with enough practice.

Kneading – You can perform this just the same way that you would knead dough. It is easy and it is recommended for the fleshy parts like the buttocks. You will have to get hold of the muscles between the thumb and the other fingers and lift gently, let go, repeat the same, press and so on. It is very relaxing, a good way to connect two lovers.

Massaging the legs – The legs are part and parcel of the Tantra massage because they are very sensitive. You should start with the long stroking massage and then caress them with the tips of your fingers. Good leg massage is best given when she is lying on her stomach.

Buttocks massage – This important body part should never be missed out in any Tantra massage book. You should proceed from the legs to the buttocks, a very erotic part of the body. This is part of, or a prelude to foreplay. As we said before, kneading and stroking are perfect techniques for this part. However, since the buttocks are fleshy, you require no kneading expertise.

Tantric Yoni Massage

One Tantra massage that every man should learn is the Yoni massage. The secret to her heart is through the Yoni (female genitals), otherwise commonly referred to as the "sacred space." Every woman worships her sexuality, and it's that connection to her sexual self that turns her from a female into a radiant goddess. What happens during the Yoni massage? You internally massage her vagina to help her achieve a full spirit experience that's sexually healing, awakening, and empowering.

This form of Tantra massage is more spiritual than it is physical, and its success largely depends on how you connect to her emotions and mental sense. A woman's sexual organs mean a lot to her physical and spiritual health. Toxins in our body systems lead to unwanted blockages, which consequently stonewall the free flow of sexual energy throughout the body. When properly done, a Yoni massage helps clear out such blockages by initiating breakdown of toxins, while at the same time increasing blood flow to her sexual organs. Before you give her the Yoni massage, make sure that the space is relaxing, and that she's absolutely comfortable.

Tips to Arouse Her

Arousing her passion and exciting her mind is an art that Tantra knows too well. This art is not just confined to touch, but a lot more. Try out these foreplay tips:

- *Kiss her neck*

Kiss the back of her neck and her ears passionately to turn her on. Some women will really be turned on when you nibble their ear lobes or lightly bite their necks.

- *Give her a foot massage*

One way that a woman achieves orgasmic bliss is through her feet. Using a high-quality moisturizer, gently massage her feet as she lies still in her bed. You may also want to tongue her feet.

- *Whisper in her ear*

Speaking softly into her ears as you cozy up in bed turns her on. Try whispering in her ears while on the phone as well.

- *Share flirty texts*

You can turn her on by simply sending her sexy texts.

- *Soft touches*

You can do this intentionally or make it look like the whole thing is outright accidental. Touch her arms or the lower back to turn her on.

- *Seduce her publicly*

Some women are easily turned on when seduced socially. Gently touch her lower back as you guide her on the sidewalk. This quickly warms up her sexual sensors.

- *Tongue her nipples*

You can do this as you massage her breasts.

- *Talk dirty*

Some women get horny when you say dirty words to them. Words like "I want to make you wet" quickly turn her on.

- *Lick her inner thighs*

Let her spread her legs, and with your tongue, taste her inner thighs.

- *Let her watch an erotic movie*

Just like men, women too are turned on by erotic movie scenes. Start with soft porn if she's comfortable with it.

- *Blindfold her*

This may not work for all women, but for some women, stealing their sense of sight helps awaken tens of other senses that you didn't know existed in the first place.

- *Vary the routine*

One way of arousing a woman is to change your sexual regimen. Don't be so predictable.

Woman Massaging Man

Woman to man tantric massage is very common. This therapy only involves massage to help with body and soul healing for sexual energy awakening. Because Tantra is the coming together of opposites, women are believed to help men release energy more easily and achieve physical, spiritual and emotional reunion faster.

What to look for in woman to man tantric massage

Women are like flowers –tender - and in some cases viewed as goddesses. Once the boundaries have been set and goals established, a man easily connects with the sexual energy awakening in Tantra sessions.

With women masseurs, the focus goes beyond simply attaining erectile health. The release of energy and spread to the entire body helps to clear tension, depression, stress and other emotional issues. When this is regularly repeated with a partner or wife at home, or simply by visiting a tantric masseur often, life takes a complete change for the better.

When the soft hands of a woman knead your muscles, you are going to experience a release of all blocked energy. With a professional female masseur, no disappointment as a spiritual route to sexual peak is achieved.

Tantric Lingam Massage

One way to help your man last longer and have better control over his sexual drive and energy is through a tantric lingam massage. So what's a lingam massage? Lingam massage is the sacred summit of a Tantra massage that combines different strokes and grip techniques on the male genitals (perineum, testicles and prostate) to help prolong his erection and delay ejaculation. It improves blood circulation throughout his body, makes erection stronger and leads to a whole-body orgasm (lasting bliss). Tantra expands our view of the lingam beyond our narrow focus on the physical. A tantric lingam massage, to a large extent, gives a woman a chance to honor and worship her partner's sexual organs. The focus is not orgasm, but to help your partner grow new sexual consciousness. Every region on the lingam (male genitals) relates to a unique body area and different energy center, hence the different pleasure zones. Each of these pleasure zones generates a unique mental state—specific physiological, psychological and emotional effect on his body system. For instance, by simply massaging his upper lingam, you can relieve his headache and, similarly, massaging the lower lingam helps relieve abdominal stress and other digestion problems. Tantric lingam massage is more spiritually beneficial and pleasurable if the man can keep a strong erection as long as his partner hasn't yet reached orgasm. The lingam enjoys a rich supply of nerve endings and caution should be taken to ensure that they're not over stimulated.

The upper side of the lingam corresponds to the man's back, while the lower side of the lingam can be likened to his front side (the face, chest, and abdomen). This shows how the lower side of the lingam is more active and sensitive compared to the lingam's upper region, which is relatively passive. Working up the upper lingam will therefore help relieve backache and of course, clean up his central channel. On the other hand, massaging the lower side helps create intimacy and activate man's emotional aspects. If a man has trouble lasting long in bed, then his woman will have trouble achieving a deep vaginal orgasm, simply because his erection has a shorter life. The different pleasure zones of his lingam should be massaged differently to achieve better results.

Tips to Arouse Him

There's a way that you can torture your man sweetly to build his anticipation. Once he's turned on, subsequent touches are just an extra delicacy. Try out these stimulation techniques to "sweet-torture" him:

- *Dance dirty for him*

Performing a slow erotic dance or something sensual for your man is a great way to turn him on. A large percentage of men will be happy to see you masturbate in their presence.

- *Tease-talk*

Just like women, men also enjoy a well-timed naughty talk. Whisper in his ears nasty lines that will turn him on. Think of over-sexualized things that you can do for him. What if you told him you didn't have your panties on? Try saying that to him in a public place.

- *Show him some booty*

Most men are turned on when they see a bit of booty. Don't shy away from showing some flesh in your lingerie. Alternatively, simply flash some unclothed breast at him or just show him something (like a tattoo), anything considered by many a taboo.

- *Touch him*

Drive his passion by touching him "inappropriately." Other than reaching out for his erogenous zones, touch his arms, neck and back as well. Grope his crotch repeatedly to get him on instantly.

- *Dress up for him*

You don't need to do much to get your man panting for you. Dress up in some tight clothes that accentuate your body, some sexy underwear, or simply show him some skin.

- *Shower with him*

Men are more of a "plug-n-play" gadget. Simply join them in the shower and they'll go with the flow.

- *Sleep naked*

Join your man in bed with nothing on. Make sure that he can feel as much of your skin as possible.

- *Reveal some thigh gap*

To bring out the sexy "triangle" simply wear some close-fitting jeans. This is a turn on for many.

- *Stare at him*

An intense eye contact is enough to make him know that there's something you can share.

Kama Sutra Sexual Handbook

It is unlikely that you have never heard of the Kama Sutra before, but you may be unfamiliar with what exactly it is. Some may think of it as simply a book of sex positions, while others may know a bit more of the history and how it came to be. Since the Kama Sutra originated in India, there are also many terms and words used throughout that you may not be familiar with, so we will make sure to breakdown some of the most commonly seen ones and provide their definitions.

With such a rich history behind it, there is so much to learn about the Kama Sutra. It is an expansive work of literature that was created to be more than just a guide on different ways in which you can have sex. Instead, it permeates all aspects of life and brings together both sexual and non-sexual ways in which you interact with a lover, a partner, or a spouse. But what exactly does "Kama Sutra" mean?

Meaning behind the Name

The word Kama is one that means pleasure but can also be translated as desire or longing. There is a sexual connotation associated with the word, meaning it is more to do with sexual pleasure and desire than with the pleasures of life or desire for material goods, but that doesn't mean that the Kama Sutra as a whole is limited to only sexual pleasure. Sutra, on the other hand, translates to verse or scripture. When you put these words together, you get the translation of "Scripture of Pleasure", but there are many variations on how you can literally translate this.

Delving deeper into the meaning behind the name, the pleasure that is Kama is one that is of all five senses, and this is very important. While many thinks of the Kama Sutra as a sex book, it is actually a book that focuses on pleasing all of the senses and is meant to be a guide on how to live a good life and enjoy yourself. From the physical enjoyment of sex to the pleasure that is derived from being in love, the Kama Sutra is filled with different verses that cover a wide range of different activities and pleasures.

While we did mention that Kama often has a sexual connotation, like with all translations there are different meanings depending on how it is being used. Kama can also be used when referencing love or affection, and in this sense, it is used in a non-sexual way. This is why the Kama Sutra needs to be viewed as a whole, since it was not intended to simply be a sexual book, but more so an erotic manual on life.

We know that the Kama Sutra extends beyond just the physical pleasures, as the book touches on the four different virtues of life.

Those four are:

- Dharma – How to live a virtuous life

- Kama – How to enjoy the pleasures of the senses

- Moksha – How to be liberated from the cycle of reincarnation

- Artha – How to gain material wealth

These four virtues are tenants of Hinduism, which is applicable since the Kama Sutra originates in India where Hinduism is one of the predominant religions. This historical context allows us to understand the book better, as we need to approach it from the mindset of the author, who would have most likely been a practicing Hindu. The author saw sexual pleasure as one of the main virtues of life, and it was both a necessary and spiritual pursuit that was important both from a non-sexual and sexual avenue. These virtues are almost instructions on how a person should live in order to be fulfilled both in this life as well as in the afterlife. Regardless of what your personal religion is, all the points are still applicable, as basic human nature dictates that we are all attempting to be the best version of ourselves and to accomplish everything we set out to gain.

Some other words that you may encounter within the Kama Sutra, and their translations, are:

- Devi – Goddess

- Gandharva – A form of marriage in which everyone is consenting to it

- Lingam – Penis

- Nayika – A woman who is desired by someone

- Prahanana – Striking or slapping someone during sex

- Raja – King

- Shlokas – Messages from above that are used to end every part of the Kama Sutra

- Vatsala – A married woman who has children

- Vikrant – A brave and beloved man

- Yoni – Vagina

Within this book, we will try and use as much of the original language as possible, so having a glossary of terms will be beneficial. With that said, however, there will always be translations available throughout so that you can follow along with ease.
So why does the literal meaning of the name even matter?

Well, understanding what an author is trying to convey is important as it allows us to enter the book and adjust our personal views so that we do not bring in our biases and preconceived notions. If you come into the Kama Sutra thinking it should only include some sex positions and nothing more, then you miss out on the richness that is contained within. Likewise, if you ignore the historical significance behind the text, you fail to grasp many of the concepts located within. In order to gain as much as you can from the Kama Sutra, you need to know what the author intended with it, and why they felt the need to create this work of literature.

History of the Kama Sutra

The exact date that the Kama Sutra was written is not known, but estimates place it anywhere between 400 BCE and 300 CE. What we do know, however, is that it was officially compiled and turned into the book that we know today in the 2nd century, otherwise known as 2 CE. This does not mean though that the book has not undergone revisions since then, and some scholars believe that the version we have is actually closely linked to the 3rd century, as some of the references throughout would not have been applicable to the 2nd century. With the text being so old, exact dating is virtually impossible, nevertheless, there is a lot of information we do know about it.
We do know that the text originates from India, although the exact location is unknown. Historians have been able to narrow down the location to somewhere within the north, or northwest, region but beyond that, it is a guess as to where the author was from. As for the author himself, we do know it was written by a man named Vatsyayana Mallanaga, as his name is engraved into the beginning of the text. Who this man was is unclear, but we do have information as to why he wrote the Kama Sutra?

Since it's compilation in the 2nd-3rd century, the Kama Sutra has undergone numerous translations and there are versions in almost every language. It was originally written in Sanskrit, an ancient Indian language, and this is the language that many Hindu scriptures were written in. While some translations are quite accurate, it is important to note that some translators did place their own bias into their work and that can be seen in the discrepancies that were later found. One of the key examples of this was in the 19th century, when the Kama Sutra was translated into English. The translator at that time wanted to ensure that the role of women in the sexual realm was not as prominent, as that was not the culture of the times. In order to maintain that societal understanding of sex and women, the Kama Sutra was altered so that women were significantly downplayed throughout. This has since been corrected, but it is important to be aware of this if you ever decide to pick up a copy for yourself as you want to be sure you are getting a purer translation.

The foundations of the Kama Sutra are rooted within the Vedic Era of literature, which is based on the word Vedas. Vedas were historical texts written in India around this time that dealt with lifestyle and how one should conduct themselves on a daily basis. All works of this time period were verbally passed down, and traditions were later adapted into many of the Hindu beliefs that are now practiced today. In the Vedic Era, there were distinct classes and castes within society, and a lot of that is reflected within the Kama Sutra. Many references are made to those who are in differing classes, and how relationships between individuals of different castes cannot work out. While this type of information is not apparently meaningful in today's culture, it does cross over when we look at socio-economic statuses and how the rich and poor interact even today.

These foundations are incredibly important because they shape the mind frame of the author of the Kama Sutra. Without grasping the history, you cannot possibly grasp what is being studied, as many of the terms and concepts no longer exist or are practiced currently.

It is with this in mind that we can start to see that the Kama Sutra is a religious text by some accounts. We may not associate sex and religion as being intertwined, but in fact, Vatsyayana saw sex as being a religious experience as well as a requirement to live a proper life. The basis of the entire viewpoint stems from certain religious beliefs, and the foundation for the entire book comes from his personal, religious beliefs. It is a celebration of human sexuality and the most carnal of pleasures, which are gifts from the gods and ultimately a necessity in life.

Philosophy of the Kama Sutra

As we said, we do know a bit about why Vatsyayana wrote the Kama Sutra. Looking at ancient Hindu texts, we know that the four virtues were commonly known and written at length about. Many of the texts focused on the two important virtues of Dharma (morality), and Athra (prosperity), while few really delved into the importance of Kama (pleasure). Vatsyayana meditated upon this reality and came to the conclusion that Kama was just as important as all of the other virtues, and so it was only proper to have a guide written solely about how to obtain Kama.

The four virtues can be looked at more as goals that each person much work towards within their lifetime in order to lead a complete and fulfilled life. Within the Kama Sutra, there are many references to the other virtues as they are all tied together and must be achieved in order to succeed. One cannot simply focus on the physical pleasures and ignore the need for morality or prosperity, so you may notice throughout that sex and morality are often combined, as well as sex and finding a partner that brings about monetary prosperity.

To understand the philosophy behind the Kama Sutra, it is vital that you understand what it was intended to be. The sex acts that are described throughout are little more than theatrics, with an emphasis on outrageous and yoga-inspired poses. The goal was unlikely to be used as a literal manual, but instead to be used as a way to understand both society and the individual. A vast majority of the book is taken up by discussing how men and women interact within society, both as a whole and simply with each other. It can be seen as almost a screenplay, taking us on a journey of love within ancient Indian times. There is talk of love, intimacy, and mundane tasks such as bathing and grooming. The Kama Sutra is a manual on all aspects of pleasure, both in the sexual sense and in the day to day realm.

Kama is so often seen as something that is less important than other aspects of human pursuit. We are told to work hard, earn money, find a spouse, have children, and live a moral and righteous life. But rarely are advised on how to let loose and enjoy ourselves, or how important of a role sex plays in the human experience. The Kama Sutra is the bridge over that gap, intended to lift up the importance of pleasure and sex, and place it in as high of regard as all the other aspects we are expected to work towards.

Some have questioned whether or not the Kama Sutra really is a female positive as it may appear, but if you approach it from the idea of the times, then it can actually be seen as more of a feminist work of art than the surface would suggest.

There is an obvious sexual freedom that is talk within, one in which even our current societal viewpoint doesn't always acknowledge. Try bringing up the topic of female masturbation and see the sudden puritanical viewpoint that many people rush to. Movies are quick to showcase men in a sexual manner, but female sexuality is much more often subdued or removed completely from the narrative. To have a book that explores the different facets of a woman's sexuality is unique both historically as well as in the current climate. Given that the Kama Sutra talks almost nothing of procreation, it truly highlights the idea that this is a guide for pleasure and nothing more. So, by its own very nature, it is also a book dedicated to a woman's pleasure, both by herself and that which is given to her by her partner. Beyond just sex, the Kama Sutra also discusses how to treat a woman properly so that she is nurtured and cared for in all aspects of life. It discusses showering her with affection and gifts and giving her absolute power when it comes to the home's finances.

From a philosophical standpoint, the Kama Sutra opens our minds to the needs of both men and women, and it does a good job of including women in the discussion, especially for the times. Not only does it take a more liberal and open-minded approach to women, but that same approach is extended to homosexuality and bisexuality as well. There are many references and discussions about men sleeping with men, and women pleasuring other women, as well as advice on having threesomes and even orgies.

The Kama Sutra makes us think by challenging our conceptions and internalized beliefs when it comes to sex. Whether it is something we partake in or not, it opens our eyes to the different forms of relationships that can exist both romantically and sexually and offers up advice on how to succeed in achieving absolute pleasure. It removes the idea that sex should be for procreating and instead emphasizes the pleasure that can be found within a sexual encounter. On a deeper level, it challenges the notion that physical pleasure should take a backseat to otherworldly pursuits, and that pleasure is just as important in life as everything else. For a life without pleasure, it isn't truly a life worth living at all.

How to Use the Kama Sutra?

The Kama Sutra can be used in two ways, both as a practical guide as well as a philosophical work of art. Some may approach the Kama Sutra only as a guide to sex positions and this is perfectly acceptable as a large chunk of text is dedicated to this pursuit. However, to use the Kama Sutra fully, you must look at it as a whole and take into account both the historical significance as well as the idea that it may not be as practical as one may originally think.

Many of the sex acts described within the Kama Sutra are outside a normal person's ability and require a high degree of flexibility to perform. There are even positions within the book that are physically impossible unless the man has a very uniquely shaped lingam (penis). Later in this book, we will look at some of the positions that are possible, however, and break down how exactly you can do them and incorporate them into your personal sex life. In many ways, there are a number of similarities between the sex acts within this book and the practice of yoga. Through breathing as one with your partner, folding into different positions, and experiencing everything in unity you can achieve a higher sense of awareness and satisfaction. So, even if you are unable to achieve the positions as described, think of it more like a workout for the mind and body and attempt a sexier form of yoga.

Since the positions are not always practical, you should use the Kama Sutra more as a general guide for how to deepen your pleasure. This book has taken many of the important concepts and ideas and broken them down into practical tips and advice so that you can elevate your sex life and truly engage in a more pleasurable and sensual experience. Beyond just the sexual side of it all, the Kama Sutra should also be used as a guide on how to treat your partner both inside and outside of the bedroom. It can assist you in being more romantic and intimate, as well as teach you how to make sure your partner is satisfied completely within the relationship.

Sex In Pregnancy

Pregnancy is the ultimate result for couples who had 1 sessions may have been a result of the urge to conceive and make a family. Most partners lose interest in sex after designing or if their partners conceive. If you suffer from the same condition, you should take measures to ensure that you do not lose interest in intimacy due to a short term condition. You may have difficulties expressing your feelings for each other due to concerns over pregnancy. It is safe to have sex during pregnancy and may be beneficial for you and the unborn. It is worth noting that there is a need to be cautious when having sex in at this time to ensure that you do not cause trouble. For that reason, you should make the following considerations for a safe and intimate session during pregnancy.

Considerations for Sex in Pregnancy

Discuss: It is an essential aspect of sex during pregnancy as the partners should be comfortable and relaxed for an intimate session. The discussion should involve the positions that you will incorporate throughout the session as well as the pace and depth of penetration. Besides, you should get a doctor's approval after doing the necessary check-ups that will give the go-ahead or make reservations.

Limitations: You should also understand the barriers that are associated with sex during pregnancy. They include keeping a low paced performance and making the session as intimate and straightforward as possible. Besides, other limitations should be observed to ensure that you do not affect the pregnancy and specifically the unborn baby. It includes avoiding combining anal sex and vaginal sex as it may lead to the transfer of bacteria.

Records: While having sex during pregnancy, you should ensure that it does not bring complication to the woman or the unborn baby. Avoid engaging in this form of sex if your partner has a history of miscarriage.

History: You must have known your partner if she is pregnant for you. For that reason, you should ensure that the activity does not affect the timing of her labor. Similarly, you should look out for the history of membrane eruption that is mostly associated with deep penetration and hard-hitting. Membrane eruption is as a result of leakages of the amniotic fluid that acts as a protector from external factors.

Cervix: You need to take your partner for a thorough check-up of the cervix to ensure that it is in the perfect condition that makes it right for sex. Ignoring this consideration may lead to other severe conditions that would require special attention from medical experts.

Positions: The big bump in pregnancy may act as a facilitator or an obstruction during sex. Therefore, you should opt for flexible positions that make it easy for both of you. The side by side rear entry position acts as a perfect example of positions that would be easy and sexually stimulating.

Make Necessary Reports: You should check on your partner every time you have sex to ensure that there are no abnormalities or straining. Make appropriate reports to the doctor if you detect problems such as pain or discharge during sex. These discharges may include blood which is a clear indication of a severe malfunction. If any of these problems in observed you should leave the sexual activity and ensure that you take necessary actions to inhibit them.

Maintain Intimacy: Regardless of the stage of pregnancy, you should maintain intimate sessions before, during, and after pregnancy. It will make it easier to resume positions even after your partner delivers. Failure to maintain intimacy after your partner conceives may lower her self-esteem and eventually lose interest in future sex. Consequently, you would require a desperate measure to rejuvenate the mood or miss it altogether.

Membrane Eruption: Deep penetration, as well as inappropriate sex positions, would lead to membrane eruption and possibly miscarriage. You should check out for signs of bleeding and pain during intercourse as warnings to these possibilities.

Pros

1. Eases labor: Frequent sex sessions make it easy for the woman to give birth and recover. The contraction of muscles experienced during sex aids in strengthening the pelvic muscles. As a result, the vagina easily opens up while resuming its previous state due to the flexibility of muscles.

2. Fewer breaks: The contractions cause muscle movements to make it easy for the vagina to hold any discharge that is associated with pregnancy. As a result, the woman can hold for long, thus requiring less time for making bathroom breaks.

3. Prevention: Engaging in sex while pregnant is beneficial for it incorporates nutrients from the sperms that aid in the growth of the unborn and the well-being of the woman. The protein found in sperms offer nutrients that help prevent pre-eclampsia.

4. Controls Blood Pressure: Sex controls your blood pressure when you are pregnant. The activity itself acts as an exercise that aids in blood circulation throughout the body, strengthening your immune system and respiration. These are essential aspects that determine your health and that of the unborn.

5. Boosts mood: It is common to experience mood swings, especially when you are pregnant. The condition worse if your partner shows no sexual expression. For that

reason, you should engage in frequent sex to maintain orgasm remain focused. Orgasm induces the circulation of blood in your pelvis, which is vital for the health of your uterus and vagina. The ripened pelvis makes it right to prepare for labor and safe delivery.

6. Improves Self-Esteem: Pregnancy comes with its effects on how you perceive yourself. The biological processes that take place during this time affect the hormonal balance hence the lowering of self-esteem. However, your partner's sexual stimulation and caressing revamp your self-confidence as you feel treasured and adored regardless of the condition.

7. Reduces Stress: The loneliness associated with pregnancy nay make a woman indulges in self-examination and worries about the unborn. The most common results are depression and stress, which could reduce through companionship and intimacy. By caring for your pregnant partner and giving her the best sexual stimulation, you reduce her stress and refresh her mind.

8. Nurtures Your Relationship: Sex during pregnancy jakes it clear that you love your partner unconditionally. They feel endowed and appreciated knowing that they hold a precious gift in them. Finding time to connect with your partner during pregnancy boost a mutual connection which soars even after conception.

Cons

1. Premature Labor: There have been cases of premature labor in couples who engage in sex during pregnancy. The cases are high, especially if the pregnancy is on the third trimester. For this reason, you should consult your doctor before engaging in sex at this period.

2. Vaginal Bleeding: The sensitivity of the pelvis makes it prone to injury, especially if the man makes a deep penetration or hits it hard. There may be excessive bleeding putting the woman at risk of low blood count, which is a severe condition in pregnancy.

3. Infections: Sex during pregnancy requires partners to be cautious about how they engage. Some practices could put both the mother and the unborn at risk of

infections. An example would be caused by combining anal sex with vaginal sex which would bring bacteria to the pelvis and eventually affect the unborn.

Except if your primary care physician reveals to you else, it is consummately alright for you to engage in sexual relations all through your pregnancy. Be that as it may, towards the normal birth date, your size may make numerous positions awkward for you. Infiltration might be least demanding if you lie on your side and your accomplice enters from behind. Oral sex and shared masturbation should cause no issues. A few ladies dread that sexual movement or climax may trigger off work yet sex can't prompt work except if the infant is expected in any case, when the prostaglandin present in the man's semen may make it start.

The sex drive of certain ladies diminishes during the primary trimester of pregnancy. This might be because of tiredness and sickness, or to a shrouded conviction that it isn't 'right' for a mother to appreciate sex. The issue will, for the most part, vanish voluntarily. In certain ladies, the sex drives increments during the center three months (the subsequent trimester) of pregnancy, and in some cases that their lovemaking is more fulfilling than any other time in recent memory. This might be because the elevated level of flowing hormones implies that a lady can be animated all the more effectively and arrive at a pitch of sexual fervor more rapidly than when not pregnant. A pregnant lady's sexual organs bosoms, areolas, and private parts - are particularly exceptionally created, which presumably increments sexual mindfulness. At last, there is finished opportunity from the stress of getting pregnant, which permits a more profound degree of 'giving up'. A few ladies and their accomplices stress that sex may hurt the unborn youngster, yet such apprehensions are baseless. The baby is shielded from disease by the attachment of bodily fluid at the neck of the belly. In uncommon cases, contamination can occur; however, this is for the most part because of the absence of typical cleanliness safety measures or engaging in sexual relations with a few unique accomplices. The infant is additionally ensured against being squashed by the amniotic liquid in which it glides in the belly. Keep away from over-athletic sex since it will be awkward for you, yet don't stress over harming the child. Sex ought not to cause premature delivery in a typical, sound pregnancy.

You can continue sex after labor when it is agreeable to do as such, ladies who have had an episiotomy (in which the perineum is sliced to encourage birth), will presumably feel sore for at any rate three weeks. At the point when you feel certain that your injury has recuperated, start to restore your sexual coexistence, taking it gradually and delicately and utilizing a greasing up jam if important to anticipate scar tissue causing uneasiness or torment.

It is essential to build up sexual contact with your accomplice when you can, as you will both need to draw near once more. On the off chance that regardless you feel sore, recollect there are different methods for giving and getting friendship. Try not to let your accomplice feel that you are showering all your consideration and consideration on your child and barring him from your affection.

Positions for pregnancy

Spoons
The lady lies serenely on her side, and the man enters her from behind, accommodating his body near hers. This position puts no weight on the lady's midriff and is reasonable for the most developed phases of pregnancy. The man can nestle very close and stroke her bosoms while kissing her shoulders and the scruff of her neck.
Leapfrog
The lady bows on the bed with legs spread wide and falls easily advances as the man enters her from behind. He would then be able to touch her back and control the profundity of push. This position is perfect when the lady begins to feel awkward with the man's weight pushing down on her, and she needs to shield her midriff from over-energetic pushing.
Astride
This is a decent position for the center a very long time of pregnancy when the teacher position has gotten awkward; however, the lady has a lot of vitality for sex. She sits on the back of the man's lap and supports herself with her arms. He can help her as she goes all over him, taking control when she gets worn out.

Conclusion

You may have started out this book confused as to why such an ancient piece of literature is still held up today as one of the most well-known books on sexual intercourse, but we hope that after reading through you have discovered much of what the Tantric sex has to offer. With such a rich and vibrant history, there is much more to the Kama Sutra than just some exotic positions, and instead, it details an entire way to live so that you can enjoy all the pleasures of life.

Living a life based on Tantric practices helps us achieve balance through the integration of feminine and masculine aspects of ourselves so that we feel a sense of wholesome that is presently lacking in our lives. Tantric practices help us see the divine in everything around us. These practices (if done patiently and diligently) infuse our senses and bodies with copious amounts of unbridled and unconditional love and compassion for one and all.

Additionally, when we practice Tantra, we are rid of baseless shame, guilt, and embarrassment associated with our sexuality that are again built around insensitive conditioning of our society. So, bringing in Tantra into your life translates to more love, compassion, and an increased sense or perception of the divine.

Tantric practices also help you use the preserved energy to find your true purpose. Of course, it is important to start small, begin with the simple individual and couple techniques mentioned in this book (which can be started immediately) and once you have mastered the simple ones and drawn the amazing benefits of even these simple tantric practices, you can move on and learn more advanced techniques from reputable teachers and take your life to an entirely new level of consciousness.

It's an exact series of steps that allow and provide to others the wellness and understanding that you should have wit yourself, and with others. As you see, Tantric sex is one of the best ways to bolster the relationship that you have with the person that you love, and if you feel like you could benefit from tantric sex, then try it.

This is a beginner's guide to understanding the power of tantra, what it is, and some of the important factors associated with this, and some of the different factors that go into tantra. The right mindset for tantra will change the way your body handles all of the different aspects of tantra, and you should understand that, with tantra, you'll feel amazing, but you should also understand that it is a powerful technique, and it can change you.

With that being said, the following step for you to take is simple. That is to try out tantric sex with your partner. You can start out small by trying out breathing and going for about ten minutes or so and work up to it. Try using tantric sex in the bedroom with some of the small techniques that are there or the positions that are associated with this. With tantra, anyone can do it, and we provided the steps for you to get started on the pathway to pleasure though this type of sex.

So, take a moment, close your eyes, and think about everything that makes you feel alive. Now, give yourself the freedom to partake in all of those pleasures, and then you will truly understand the power of the Tantric Sex.